Modern Approach to Colposcopic Findings

Atlas for the Practitioner in Gynaecology

By

Dr. med. ULRICH BERGMANN

73 plates

AKADEMIE-VERLAG · BERLIN

1982

Published by Akademie-Verlag, GDR - 1086 Berlin, Leipziger Str. 3—4
Proof editor: Christiane Grunow

Licence No.: 202 · 100/531/82
Composited and printed by VEB Druckhaus „Maxim Gorki“, 7400 Altenburg, GDR
Order No.: 763 015 7 (6650) · LSV 2715/2145
Printed in GDR
DDR 58,— M

Prefatory Note

The complete route of canceration in the cervix uteri, including facultatively phased-out canceration, the phases being dysplasia, carcinoma in situ, microcarcinoma, and ordinary carcinoma, has been a discovery in gynaecological research of the utmost importance to clinical and theoretical oncology.

Hans *Hinselmann* and his students, with ingenious concepts, had been the first to perceive from the cervix model cancer in this totality.

The use of the colposcopic magnifying glass in tracing carcinogenetic processes in the cervix will remain to be an integral component of cancer research, the more as carcinogenesis can be associated today with an oncogenically infectious nucleoproteid.

Ulrich *Bergmann* has been extremely successful in presenting brilliant modern documentation as an introduction to this kind of colposcopy.

March, 1979 W. *Eschbach*, Berlin-Buch

Foreword

A renaissance of colposcopy is now being experienced by gynaecologists all over the world, with magnifier-tracing of carcinogenesis, with emphasis on the vascular aspect, assuming ever more importance.

This "Modern Approach to Colposcopic Findings" has been written and compiled with particular attention being given to that vascular aspect, for all who are interested in learning more about the variety of benign and malignant neoplasias, inflammations, and regenerative processes.

Black-and-white film was deliberately used for photographic documentation, since the author and his colleagues feel that in modern colposcopy the vascular picture has to be the decisive criterion for colposcopic diagnosis. A 6×6 camera was used for negative magnification of 1 to 3 and print magnification up to a factor of 25. Attached to it was an Apogerminar 140 mm close-up lens by Kombinat Carl Zeiss Jena (GDR) and an annular flash. This is the proper place to pay tribute to Herr *Wotzka*, the photographer, for the excellent job he has done.

The photographic plates of this Atlas were prepared in the Gynaecological Section of Robert-Rössle-Klinik, an institution of the GDR Academy of Sciences, Central Institute of Cancer Research.

I am under a particular debt of gratitude to Prof. Dr. med. habil. Walter *Eschbach*, Medical Superintendant of the Gynaecological Section in the Central Institute of Cancer Research. Being my distinguished academic teacher, he has introduced me to *Hinselmann's* colposcopy and to his own successfully treated subject, facultatively phased-out canceration in the cervix uteri, induced by an oncogenically infectious nucleoproteid.

An expression of cordial gratitude goes to Akademie-Verlag, GDR - 1080 Berlin, represented by Christiane *Grunow*, the proof editor, and Klaus *Todten*, the make-up editor. With great personal commitment, devotion, and high professional skill, they have made valuable contributions to making this project reality.

A word of particular appreciation must be extended to Wolfgang *Ghantus* who has spared no pains in producing an excellent English translation of this Atlas.

Finally, recognition is deserved also by the personnel of VEB Druckhaus „Maxim Gorki", GDR-7400 Altenburg, who have accomplished a highly satisfactory production of both text and illustrations.

Dr. med. Ulrich *Bergmann*
Specialist in Gynaecology and Obstetrics
1115 Berlin-Buch, GDR
Hobrechtsfelder Chaussee 100

Contents

EDITORIAL SECTION

Comments on terminology

Hinselmann's classical colposcopic terminology is used in the text of this Atlas. The author felt encouraged to do so because of historic aspects, as *Hinselmann's* first pacemaking findings in the field of colposcopy were revealed to the public, more than 50 years ago. Yet, the author also felt a need for suggesting that the variety of colposcopic findings, including the relative importance of canceration phases, is very conditionally reflected in the terminology adopted by FIGO in 1975. The FIGO terms are given in parentheses in the headlines of the text but placed at the beginning of the plate captions.

Colposcopic terminology adopted by FIGO, 1975:

A. Normal colposcopic findings

1. Original squamous epithelium
2. Columnar epithelium
3. Transformation zone

B. Abnormal colposcopic findings

1. Atypical transformation zone
   a) Mosaic
   b) Punctuation
   c) White epithelium
   d) Keratosis
   e) Atypical vessels
2. Suspect frank invasive carsinoma

C. Unsatisfactory colposcopic findings (squamocolumnar junction not visible)

D. Miscellaneous colposcopic findings

1. Inflammatory changes
2. Atrophic changes
3. Erosion
4. Condyloma
5. Papilloma
6. Etc.

Normal colposcopic findings:

1. Original squamous epithelium — is a smooth, pink, and featureless epithelium originally established on the cervix and vagina. There are no remnants of columnar epithelium identified, such as mucous secreting epithelium, cleft openings or Nabothian cysts.

2. Columnar epithelium — is a single layer mucus producing tall epithelium which extends between the endometrium cranially and either the original squamous epithelium or the metaplastic epithelium caudally. Area covered with columnar epithelium has irregular surface with long stromal papillae and deep clefts. In the colposcope, after acetic acid test, it has a typical grape-like structure. Columnar epithelium may be present in the endocervix, on the portio or even in the vagina.

3. Transformation zone — is the area between original squamous epithelium and columnar epithelium in which metaplastic epithelium in varying degrees of maturity is identified. Components of a normal transformation zone may be islands of the columnar epithelium surrounded by metaplastic squamous epithelium, "gland openings", and Nabothian cysts. In normal transformation zones there are no colposcopic findings suggestive of cervical neoplasia.

Abnormal colposcopic findings:

1. Atypical transformation zone — is a transformation zone in which there are colposcopic findings suggestive of cervical neoplasia.

a) Mosaic — is a focal abnormal colposcopic lesion in which the tissue has a mosaic pattern. The fields of the mosaic are separated by reddish borders.

b) Punctuation — is a focal abnormal colposcopic pattern in which the capillaries appear as a stippled pattern.

c) White epithelium — is a focal abnormal colposcopic pattern seen after acetic test. White epithelium is a transient phenomenon which is seen in the area of increased nuclear density.

d) Keratosis — is a focal colposcopic pattern in which hyperkeratosis or parakeratosis is present and appears as elevated whitened plaque. This whitened plaque is identified before application of acetic acid. At times, keratosis may be identified outside the transformation zone.

e) Atypical vessels — constitute a focal abnormal colposcopic pattern in which the blood vessel pattern appears not as punctuation, mosaic or as delicately branching vessels, but rather as irregular vessels with abrupt courses appearing as commas, corkscrew capillaries or spaghetti-like forms.

2. Suspect frank invasive cancer — is colposcopically obvious invasive cancer which is not evident on clinical examination.

Unsatisfactory colposcopic findings:

These are cases in which the squamocolumnar junction cannot be visualised.

Other colposcopic findings:

1. Inflammatory changes — constitute a diffused colposcopic pattern of hyperaemia in which the blood vessels may appear in a diffused stiplet pattern similar to the vascular pattern in punctuation.

2. Atrophic changes — are recordable from oestrogen-deprived squamous epithelium in which the vascular pattern is more readily identitied to the relative thinness of the overlying squamous epithelium.

3. Erosion — is an area denuded of epithelium, usually by trauma.

4. Condyloma and papilloma — are exophytic lesions which may be inside or outside the transformation zone.

1. General

Colposcopy had been inaugurated as a method of early carcinoma detection by Prof. Dr. med. Dr. med. h. c. Hans *Hinselmann* (6. 8. 1884—18. 4. 1959), more than 50 years ago. The method is now undergoing a period of renaissance, since *Hinselmann* succeeded in making a discovery never repeated so far in any other specialised oncological discipline of human medicine.

In an attempt to detect the smallest identifiable carcinoma, he managed to come across the preliminary stages of carcinoma of the cervix which now is considered the model carcinoma of spontaneous canceration in man.

He displayed a sense of untiring diligence, exactitude, and minute meticulosity on all his findings, in terms of thorough colposcopic and histological evaluation. He was just as active in publicising his results, with the view to making his discoveries accessible to the largest possible community of the profession. People continue to be amazed even today with his findings represented in water-colour paintings.

Unfortunately, however, colposcopy proved very slow in gaining ground, which applied also to the region of the author's own German-language tradition. *Hinselmann*, dealing successfully with strong resistance offered to him by scholarly medicine, and pathologists, in particular, succeeded, by persistent research effort and scientific publicity, in giving systematic treatment to his empirically recorded visual criteria of phased-out canceration on the portio uteri. True, many formal-genetic and causative-genetic correlations and implications have remained unelucidated to this day, but valuable images have been gained of canceration processes and their interaction with defence mechanisms of the organism as well as with processes of regulation, dysregulation, and counter-regulation.

Today, both the practitioner and the research worker have at their disposal three visual approaches based on experience which provide information on the actual degree of canceration. They are colposcopy, cytology, and histology.

Colposcopy enables evaluation, on the basis of the examiner's own experience, of objectively existing visible criteria.

Cytology enables definition of canceration phases from individual cells by means of quantitative and qualitative criteria.

Histology enables evaluation of canceration processes by relating them to surrounding tissue.

While it is quite common to define classical colposcopy as well as classical cytology as search methods and to concede the rank of a genuine diagnostic method to histology only, the point has to be made that a high diagnostic information potential must be attributed to modern differentiated colposcopy and to an even greater extent to differential cytology.

Either method is somewhat burdened with a certain error rate. With colposcopy, for example, it is impossible to achieve visual inspection of the upper two thirds of the endocervical canal. However, by combining the two methods precursor phases and early stages of carcinoma of the cervix can be diagnosed nearly with mathematical accuracy.

Colposcopy, today, enables differentiation of physiological and pathophysiological findings as well as detection, control, and monitoring of suspect changes, including carcinoma, in the region of the portio and in the lower third of the cervix. It actually offers the following benefits:

- Assessment, differentiation, and classification of physiological and pathophysiological findings;
- Localisation of the highest atypical point, as the point of departure from which to launch definite diagnostic action;
- Assessment of therapeutic interventions and post-therapeutic follow-up;
- Assessment of changes during menstruation, gravidity and with the patient on hormonal contraceptives;
- Assessment of physiological and pathophysiological processes in vagina and vulva.

2. Fundamentals of colposcopy

Colposcopy had been devised by *Hinselmann* as a method by which to diagnose earliest portio carcinomas, under the assumption that they were small and smallest tumours.

The new method revealed soon that two-dimensional intra-epithelial changes were phases precedent of carcinoma. *Hinselmann* defined those findings by coining the term of "matrix regions".

As a side-effect or by-product, so to say, of the above insight, colposcopy proved to be extremely important to improving clinical diagnosis of portio changes under a variety of physiological conditions.

2.1. Technical conditions

Physically, colposcopy may be defined as the use of a magnifying glass for stereoscopic inspection of the portio, using alternative luminous intensities and magnification factors between 7 and 35.

The optical parameters and convenient handling are the two major criteria by which a given colposcope is chosen.

A spacing of something between 22 cm and 25 cm should be allowed between the front lens of the colposcope and the portio, to enable the use of instruments without obstruction of visual inspection. The use of several magnification factors should be made possible for each given case, since the diameter of the field of vision is likely to decline along with growth in magnification factors.

The depth of field, that is the distance between two different points on the optical axis which are visible in unequal focus, will decline along with decrease in magnification. Illumination should be about 30,000 Lux, and the light source should be centered.

Colour filters may be required and, therefore, should be available together with the gadgetry to use them.

Halogen and, even better, ultraviolet light may be desirable for optimum inspection of vascular criteria.

The tripod should be designed to convenient handling and observation by the gynaecologist, and it should be easily movable in three planes.

Commercially available gynaecological chairs are good enough for examination under normal conditions. The patient should be in comfortable position.

2.2. Implementation of colposcopy

Use of the bivalve speculum has proved to enable optimum adjustment of the portio. The posterior valve is inserted in rectangular direction relative to the vaginal cleft and moved inside to a point in front of the portio.

The anterior valve is used for further unfolding of the vagina, which enables the posterior valve to be moved further, under visual control, right into the posterior fornix, without causing injury to the portio.

The anterior valve now is handed to an assisting nurse or, in an exceptional situation, even to the patient. The posterior valve is held by the examiner. In a routine check, the first colposcopic inspection should follow now. Then, a cytological smear is taken. Mucus, exudate or other matter are carefully swabbed and visually checked. Physiological saline solution may be applied to the portio, as suggested by the Oslo working group, before a first description is attempted, with emphasis being laid on the vessels.

Now, acetic acid in concentrations between two and three per sent is applied to the portio surface, which should be done best by means of a properly soaked swab. Inspection and recording of findings are followed by an attempt for deepest possible inspection of the endocervical canal.

Various techniques have been recommended for cervix unfolding, from the use of a cotton carrier to special opening, for better assessment of endocervical lesions, polypi or of the upper boundary of atypical epithelia.

Examination of the cervix must be followed, naturally, by a check of the vagina, which is accomplished by withdrawal, under colposcopic control, of the specula up to the vulva. Only now, *Schiller's* test will follow, and its result together with the colposcopic findings will form the background against which a decision may be taken for special exploratory excision.

Diagnostic palpation will complete this set of examinations. The findings obtained from any colposcopic examination should be carefully entered into the patient's file. The gynaecologist will not be in a position to realise alterations nor to carry out follow-up checks unless high-continuity documentation is available.

A drawn diagram may be best suitable for keeping findings under permanent control. There are different forms of representation for documentation between which a choice can be made to facilitate work. The properly developed and printed colpophotograph is thought to be the optional tool to keep track of pathological findings.

While this technique is irreplaceable in education and research, there has been little chance so far for its general introduction to practice.

2.3. Timing of colposcopy

No colposcopy should be used during menstruation nor between three and four days after it. Menstrual blood would inflict maceration on the squamous epithelium and, consequently, blur real lesions. Colposcopy can be most easily and safely applied, while the cervical mucous plug is flocculent and clear, with the outer foramen gaping. While transparent mucous acts like a refractory medium, opacity will cause problems for the examiner. The menstruation calendar, therefore, should be consulted for optimum timing.

2.4. Anatomic foundations of the colposcopic approach

Colposcopy, for unambiguous results, depends on assessment of the epithelium (multilayer squamous or columnar epithelium) and of the connective tissue underneath. The colposcopic picture is generated by the condition as well as by physiological and pathological changes of the epithelium, including changes attributable to substances applied by the examiner, and by vascularisation of connective tissue.

Here is a brief listing of some terms especially used in colposcopic parlance. The *ectocervix* (portio) is the region which becomes visible on speculum examination. The *endocervix* is a region which will not be visible on speculum examination unless higher technical skill is applied.

Clinically, the *external os uteri* is the very point from which the epithelium of the endocervical canal begins to extend for the purpose of speculum examination. The anatomic external os uteri can be localised only by means of anatomic examination.

The *boundary* between *columnar epithelium* and *squamous epithelium* is the line at which the monolayer columnar epithelium abuts on the multilayer squamous epithelium. That line is rarely identical with the external os uteri.

That divergence between clinical and

anatomic definition of the external os uteri results from a relative instability of the epithelial boundary which undergoes changes throughout one life span.

The *uterine cervix* is developed throughout life. It is modified by gravidity, childbirth, surgery, but mainly by age. Studies into the anatomic external os uteri have shown the columnar-squamous epithelia boundary to be located ectocervically in young women, but endocervically in women in the menopause.

The position of the labia of the os uteri is changed also, when the clinical examiner separates the vaginal vault. The clinical external os uteri then will differ from its normal position, in that it gets somewhat displaced into the endocervical canal.

Clinical examination will hardly cause any change to an external os uteri which is round and small. The anatomic and clinical pictures often are even congruent in such cases. Such picture may be recordable from nulliparae and women in the menopause. The divergence between clinical and anatomic definition of the os uteri can be extremely large in women in whom it is widely opened transversally, as may be the case with pluriparae or following complicated delivery. Many explanations have been offered for such divergence in numerous discussions, in that context.

Definition of the "external os uteri" so far is not sufficiently precise for equally unambiguous clinical and anatomic determination. The stroma of the uterine cervix is made up of tough trusswork of tissue fibres, interspersed with numerous vessels and lymphatic channels. The squamous epithelium is roughly 0.5 mm in height. Its lower surface is indented by conjunctively vascular axes which form papillae. Normally, the epithelium is stratified, consisting of something between 15 and 20 cellular layers. The columnar epithelium is formed by one single columnar cell layer with basal nucleus. Its thickness is about 0.1 mm. There are flattened cells among them, reserve cells, so to say, which play an important role in regeneration and indirect metaplasia.

The mucous menbrane is not smooth at all, but structured with deep vertical furrows and invaginated into the stroma, and so numerous "glands" are formed in the endocervical canal.

Columnar epithelium on the portio covers the connective tissue papillae, being shaped with broad base and rounded tip. Each of these papillae has one central vascular axis running through it.

The columnar-squamous epithelium boundary has some peculiarities in the vicinity of "glands", where the squamous epithelium is thinner and poor with glycogen.

The squamous epithelium stands out between 0.2 mm and 0.3 mm over the glandular epithelium. Two levels are thus produced to make the boundary easily visible.

2.5. Methods of differentiated (extended) colposcopy

Acetic acid, in concentrations of two or three per cent, has been one of the first substances used in colposcopy. Advantage is taken of its major effect, that is to cause coagulation of the cytoplasmatic nuclear proteins of the epithelium and to cause their discoloration to grey. Coagulation is progressive, superficial, reversible, and reproducible. Squamous epithelium, abnormally burdened with protein, is progressively turned grey and, finally, vinegar-white after something between ten and thirty seconds.

Alteration appears to have occurred only to superficial cells, followed, histologically, by retraction and flattening up to one third of the squamous epithelium. The same coagulative effect was found to occur also in the second half of the menstrual cycle in viscous and opaque cervical mucus.

Acetic acid has no effect at all on spinnable, mucoflocculent, clear mucus, with neither transparence nor viscosity being affected.

Yet, acetic acid has exhibited rapid and extremely impressive action upon columnar epithelium. Small greyish-white "grapes" were found to be typical features of papillary columnar epithelium. Ectopic islands can be clearly visualised in a transformation zone. Clear mucus is quite often discharged from the "glandular openings", and the latter seem to widen. However, changes which have occurred to columnar epithelium are not fully reversible, and the tissue appears to be swollen two or three days. Hence, the acetic acid test (*Hinselmann*) is a procedure by which to delimit normal squamous epithelium from normal columnar epithelium. Differentiation is equally possible between vinegar-white epithelium, metaplastic epithelium, dysplastic epithelium, and carcinoma tissue. Whitening often is helpful in strengthening the contrast between vessels and sub-base. Vascular contours, however, may be less clear or even fade away for vessels in comparatively deep position, that is under several cellular layers. The iodine test was inaugurated by *Schiller*, 1928, after he had found that little or no glycogen was contained in pathologically altered squamous epithelia.

For *Schiller's* test, the portio has to be brush-painted with Lugol's solution (iodine-iodine-potassium). Normal squamous epithelium then will turn brown, while glycogen-free epithelium will remain, practically, unstained. The following concentration is usually chosen: 2.0 of pure iodine, 4.0 of potassium with iodine, and 100.0 of distilled water. The portio has to be swabbed and painted, using a gauze swab adequately soaked with the above solution. Unfortunately, the amount of reliability expected by *Schiller* has never been reached. Yet, benefit may be obtained from subsequent diagnosis of normal glycogen-holding epithelium. Absence of iodine coloration will merely suggest absence of mature, glycogen-holding squamous epithelium.

Absence of coloration may be an indicator to the presence of dysplastic or carcinomatous or highly atrophic squamous epithelium or columnar epithelium or to the absence of epithelium at all. *Schiller's* test is very important to deciding the angle of incision for conisation.

Fine network-like or punctiform patterns may occasionally be identified from mature transformation zones by intensive inspection of the portio, following *Schiller's* test. The presence of Naboth's ovules may be another reason why staining often is reduced. Annular, poorly stained edges often are formed around "glandular" openings in a transformation zone (*Hinselmann* et al.).

Both leucoplakia (keratosis) and ectopy will regularly remain unstained. The colposcopic image may be somewhat blurred by iodine droplets which may adhere to mucus. Dysplasia may be recognised by a whitish shade, with the transformation zone often being tinted yellowish. Stippled rather than regular yellowish coloration often may be recorded after childbirth or in the postclimacteric period.

Stainability may be reduced to small whitish stippling in the presence of inflammatory processes. Yet, a distinct borderline between normal and pathological epithelium is one of the most conspicuous signs of inflammation and does not occur in a transformation zone without any pathological change.

The above methods and techniques of colposcopy have become routine practice. Yet, countless additional methods have been devised, in the course of time, their usefulness being differently rated by various authors (*Majewski* et al.). Great importance has been recently assumed by colposcopy in no-red and ultraviolet light, since in differentiated colposcopy more attention is being given to vascular criteria (*Hinselmann* et al.). Ultraviolet colposcopy has been used by *Hinselmann* also in conjunction with most various fluorescent substances.

Nevertheless, direct visual inspection of vessels, following rinsing in physiological saline solution, has come most strongly to the fore, in our days (*Kolstad, Koller, Johannisson, Söderberg*).

With no-red light, the use of a green filter (*Kraatz*) has to be considered as an intermediate stage which offers the great advantage of minimised effort. Very good inspection of vessels is possible also in halogen light which is used in modern colposcopes.

The technological solution of infrared radiation (*Menken*) as a possible approach to colpophotography appears to be relatively expensive and, consequently, not applicable to routine colposcopy and colpophotography. More importance, no doubt, will be assumed by vasostimulants, particularly for assessment of vascular criteria.

3. Normal colposcopic findings

Comprehensive knowledge of the normal colposcopic picture is absolutely essential to detection of pathological developments. The portio offers a colourful variety of images which have remained to be subdivided by three groups (*Hinselmann*).

Particularly impressive images were found to be recordable from the sexually mature woman. Generally, normal colposcopic findings are recordable by the following percentual proportionality:

> Between ten and 15 per cent from the original portio;
> Between 15 and 20 per cent from ectopy (columnar epithelium);
> Between 65 and 70 per cent from the transformation zone.

In modern colposcopy, overall assessment depends strongly on the visualised vascular pattern. Therefore, a brief account will be given of all knowledge so far gained of the fine structure of the peripheral vessels system in the cervix uteri. The account will be given, basically, with reference to the findings of *Zinser* and *Rosenbauer*.

Blood is supplied to the cervix uteri through the uterine and vaginal arteries, with the fixed point of the two blood supply regions actually being formed by the borderline between the squamous and columnar epithelia. Fibres and vessels, in a histological specimen, will always be orientated towards the "terminal cervix gland". The ascending branch of the uterine artery supplies blood to that part of the cervix which is covered with columnar epithelium, while those parts of the portio which are covered with squamous epithelium receive their blood supplies from the cervicovaginal branch of the uterine artery and from the vaginal artery. The entire ectocervix is more or less regularly interspersed with vessels. A zone with a small amount of vessels is located in the connective tissue nucleus.

The above principle of vascular supply retains its validity even for cases in which the boundary between squamous and columnar epithelia does not coincide with the external os uteri. The vessels in the stroma covered with columnar epithelium are of a stockade structure. Radial blood streams branch off from regularly spaced points of vessels which are annularly distributed around the uterine cervix, and these blood streams radiate in direction of the endocervical canal. In the lower part of the cervix, they fan out with growing steepness in direction of the external os uteri. The calibres of these vessels are smaller than those of other vessels which branch off the vaginal artery. These are strongly bifurcated and of meandering configuration.

The vascular system of the vaginal sector consists of a deep vascular plexus of horizontal alignment in the peripheral region of the ectocervix. Bifurcating from that vascular system are stockade-type vessels which end in a subpapillary grid of basal vessels. Capillaries embedded in connective tissue papillae shoot from that grid or network of basal vessels, and their terminal vessel loops stand out in differentiated density and angles, in vertical or oblique position, to reach the squamous epithelium. The papillary vessels should be colposcopically visible, under normal conditions, and so may be the basal vessels under certain circumstances.

Two basic types of capillaries, which may be present in parallel or separately, can be observed beneath normal squamous epithelium:

Network capillaries constitute one of these types. They may be found primarily in the presence of scarcely developed stromatic papillae and tend to form a high-density mesh system. Mesh spacing is smaller than the intercapillary distance of the hairpin vessels.

The second type is made up of *hairpin capillaries*. Their ascending and descending branches are spaced closely by one another to form a soft vascular arch. These capillaries usually are located in the stromatic papillae. The entire vascular arch can be colposcopically observed, provided that the surface epithelium is not too thick, but of normal transparency, while a favourable angle of inspection should be chosen, as well. However, only the crests of the vascular arch will often be visible as regularly and densely arranged small spots.

3.1. Original portio

The portio "ab origine" (*Hinselmann*) may be recorded primarily from post-menopause women, but ten per cent of such findings are recordable from women in sexual maturity.

The most common picture, by colposcopic inspection, consists of smooth, sometimes granulated, squamous epithelium of pale pink colour, usually with some light grey added. That smooth or papillary surface relief, normally, is sprinkled with clear secretion which reflects incident light.

The colour of the colposcopic image will depend on the given condition of stromatic blood flow as well as on thickness and translucency of the epithelium. In the presence of inflammatory processes, predominant shades will be red, while darker and bluish red tends to be caused by venous congestion during gravidity. With women in the menopause, the colposcopic picture tends to be discoloured yellowish to grey, because of the colour of atrophic stroma against the background of poorer blood flow. Hence, under normal conditions, the colposcopic image will be the substrate of observation of the cervical stroma with its terminal vessel paths, all covered 0.5 mm with stratified squamous epithelium. The strongly vascularised stroma with its vessels will show more or less clearly through the epithelium, depending on the latter's thickness. Careful colposcopic inspection will reveal through the epithelium either hairpin capillaries of the stroma or fine network capillaries. There may be mixed appearences as well, or vessels branching as in a tree (*Kolstad*). Spacings between hairpin capillaries are between 50 μm and 200 μm. In other cases, there may be network capillaries spaced between 50 μm and 100 μm. The squamous epithelium in five per cent of women in sexual maturity and with original portio will be stratified to thickness levels through which no vessels at all will be visible.

It has beeen one of the conspicuous findings that in sexual maturity vessels in higher or lower papillae reach into the epithelium, whereas the boundary between squamous epithelium and connective tissue and, consequently, the borderline of the capillary network practically will form a straight line beyond the age of 55.

Highly atrophic epithelium may render visible, in addition to the network capillaries, the network of basal vessels with anastomotic vessels in spiderweb arrangement (*Kos*), either mossy or with root-like contours (*Zinser*). Petechia, caused by vulnerability of both epithelium and vessels, usually is one of the additional findings.

Cervical stroma in pregnant women tends to undergo considerable congestion and discoloration to violet. The squamous epithelium will be thickened, and the network of terminal vessels will be changed, as well. Capillary loops are likely to emerge from subepithelial capillary network to form papillae for variegated penetration of epithelium. The ends of those loops are shaped like forks, trees or glomerules (*Mikolas*). The findings recordable from women on hormonal contraceptives are similar to those established from women in gravidity.

Inflammatory processes were found to cause some striking changes to the terminal section of the vascular system. Loops or spiral-shaped capillaries were found to grow out of the capillary network to penetrate the epithelium (*Kos*). The crests of those capillary loops appear colposcopically as numerous red stiplets. Some of them may be similar to diplococci by microscopic inspection. The patterns usually are regular and diffused, without clearcut demarcation line, sometimes of focal arrangement. Special attention was given to studying trichomonal colpitis (*Johannisson, Kolstad, Holtorff*). Various degrees of inflammatory severity exhibited densely arranged hairpin capillaries with double crests (double capillaries) or of cloverleaf shape.

Senile colpitis is a special form of inflammation. The subepithelial network is readily visible through the thinned epithelium (*Kolstad*). Intercapillary distance does not exceed 200 μm. Severe inflammation will be accompanied by non-persistent regressive vasodilatation, somewhat reminiscent of changes which are known under the name of papillary floor (punctuation) (*Ganse*). Conspicuous vessels may be seen also in the wake of radium irradiation or X-irradiation. These are teleangiectasias which have replaced originally carcinomatous vessels and are considered signs of favourable prognosis (*Rieck, Ganse*). Squamous epithelium of normal stratification was found to be of relatively high resistance. It will hardly change its own appearance in response to three-per-cent acetic acid and rarely show subtle whitish discoloration (*Glatthaar*).

Epithelium to which Lugol's solution is applied will turn deep-brown and iodine-positive due to the action of intracellular glycogen (*Schiller*). With atrophic epithelium, such discoloration may be towards light iodine, that is very slight, since the glycogen level is hormonally controlled. Subtle whitish punctuation usually will be recordable from the iodine-positive and iodine-brightness areas in the papillary region.

3.2. Ectopy (columnar epithelium)

"Ectopy" of columnar epithelium, i.e. occurrence of cervical epithelium at unusual points on the portio surface, may be recorded from something between ten and 15 per cent of all women, mainly young women and others in sexual maturity. In roughly 90 per cent of all cases, it is likely to undergo regression through the transformation zone.

The contact line between columnar and squamous epithelia is situated on the outer surface of the portio where it may, sometimes, form papillary outgrowths and "glands". Ectopy, according to *R. Meyer*, is the first curative phase of erosion. According to other authors (*Matejka, Ober, Hamperl*), the case may be congenital, acquired, physiological, ontogenetic, traumatic, hormonal or inflammatory ectropion.

The colposcopic image of ectopy may be that of a brilliant red surface generated by strongly vascularised stroma which shines through the monolayer columnar epithelium and may be differentiated, even macroscopically, from the more palish surrounding squamous epithelium. This is defined as erythroplakia. The smooth, reflecting surface ot the original portio has been replaced by an area of small rounded convexities. Levels are staggered 0.4 mm, and such visible staggering together with a strong red coloration have led to the definition of pseudo erosion.

Mucus secretion from this epithelium is often so strong that patients would complain about fluor (*Jakob*). The monolayer columnar epithelium is highly vulnerable, and bleeding may be caused even by swabbing The most impressive colposcopic picture of ectopy has been obtained after swabbing with acetic acid of concentrations between two and three per cent. Acetic acid causes columnar epithelium to undergo whitish discoloration and swelling. The stromatic papillae assume the appearance of "small grapes", and large amounts of transparent cervical mucus are often secreted. Those small grapes may be of rounded, regular shape or somewhat lengthened in certain cases or much larger, polypous, and of tough papillary appearance in others. The mesh net of ectopic vessels, according to *Kolstad*, is narrower than that of the original portio. Each of the small grapes has a capillary loop on its own axis. In the thin and drawn-out grapes, those capillary loops are almost reminiscent of hairpins and, therefore, often may be deceptive to the unexperienced examiner who has not used the acetic acid test.

Capillary trees, differentiated in shape, often may be detected in small grapes of tough papillary appearance. The thickness of capillaries with smooth vascular wall is conspicuously level and gives the impression of calm blood flow. In pregnancy, columnar epithelium of ectopy will turn plastic and bulging (*Sebek*). The vascular pattern is conspicuous, because of strong vascularisation, but it remains to be in line with the intensified pattern of terminal vessels on the papillary tips of ectopy.

Columnar epithelium would not be stained by *Schiller's* iodine test, as it is iodine-negative. Some authors have resorted to the argentum test, using argentum nitricum in three per cent concentration, to rule out "erosio vera".

The manifestations of ectopy can be highly variable, with deviation from the typical pattern being recordable under the following conditions:

— A squamous epithelium defect is rapidly grown over by columnar epithelium. Hence, the typical grape structure is not formed, and a false impression is given of the presence of erosio vera.

— The stroma is acutely or chronically irritated, and stromatic girders or columns are formed with papillary hypertrophy. Fine-papillary, tough-papillary or polypous ectopy are some of the definitions coined in literature to describe such patterns.

— In gravidity, often paralleled by concomitant inflammation (*Ganse*), papillae may undergo voluminous swelling due to congestion of stroma. They will then stand together in groups, the latter being separated by grooves.

Ectopy, with all its manifestations, is a temporary condition. Sooner or later will the ectocervix be covered again with squamous epithelium. This process of conversion is colposcopically represented by the picture of the transformation zone.

3.3. Transformation zone

This definition, coined by *Hinselmann*, is to describe the process by which the floor of ectopy, that is stroma of columnar epithelium, is covered with squamous epithelium.

Attempts to elucidate the genesis of "erosion", "pseudo erosion", and "healing" of such changes have been undertaken for more than 80 years by authors of outstanding renown, among them *R. Meyer*, *Hinselmann*, *Lax*, *Schottländer*, *Fischel*, *Ruge-Veit*, *Adler*, *Hamperl*, *Kaufmann*, *Ober*, *Schneppenheim*, *Clara*, *Ludwig*, *Fluhmann*, *Stoeckel*, *Schröder*, *Treite*, *Mestwerdt*, *Wespi*, *Coppleson*, *Linsbach*, *Glatthaar*, *Zinser*, *Gottschalk*, *Rosenbauer*, *Bajardi*, *Beato*, *Castaño*, *Barcellos*, *Linhartova*, and *Skolovski*. The following findings seem to bear relevance to interpretation of colposcopic patterns of the transformation zone:

— Advancing growth of squamous epithelium, from edge to centre, on top of or underneath columnar epithelium and possible proliferation of islands of squamous epithelium to overgrow columnar epithelium (*R. Meyer*);

— Metaplastic formation of squamous epithelium from the basal layer (*Ruge*);

— Vertical growth of glands and, from these, displacement of squamous epi-

thelium by columnar epithelium and, in a second phase, re-incorporation of squamous epithelium, by growth from edge to centre, and of islands of squamous epithelium which had been spared (*Schottländer, Gottschalk*);
- Overlapping of damage to cells of columnar epithelium with construction of squamous epithelium through basal cells (*Hinselmann*);
- Metaplastic alteration of basal layer and formation of new squamous epithelium in the form of regenerative metaplasia (*Fischer, Wasells*) or of prosoplasia (*Fluhmann*).

Generally, the concept of metaplastic transformation has been accepted. Metaplastic transformation has been typical of all tissues in the process of regeneration. Transformations of that kind are mostly caused by long-lasting abnormal, functional, mechanical, inflammatory, hormonal, nervous, and chemical stimuli (*Linsbach*). Hence, transformation is found to be accompanied by a process of appositioned advancing growth, from edge to centre, of squamous epithelium and of resting islands of squamous epithelium. Ploughing undergrowth and detachment of columnar epithelium and coverage of connective tissue papillae with squamous epithelium may be consequences.

Islands of columnar epithelium may continue to exist in the crypt "glands". As long as those islands of columnar epithelium retain their mucus-secretory function, "glandular openings" with outflow of clear secretion will be visible in the transformation zone. Overgrowth of those openings, with oestrogen-induced mucus secretion continued, results in the formation of cysts, Naboth's ovules. They may contain solid, stratified mucus, with their strata corresponding to menstrual cycles.

Also, squamous epithelium, usually formed in the vicinity of vessels, is likely to develop from subcolumnar reserve cells of columnar epithelium by metaplasia in the transformation zone.

Such overgrown squamous epithelium which replaces columnar epithelium should not be equalled to or confused with squamous epithelium of the original portio.

Secondary squamous epithelium is formed on connective tissue stroma of ectopic columnar epithelium. *Hinselmann* defined it as "membrane sui generis", between ectopy and original portio mucus membrane. The same, morphologically independent, tissue structure was defined as "third membrane" by *Beato* and co-workers.

The processes of transformation, regeneration, repair, and proliferation, tend to take place at too high rates for the young, usually metaplastic, squamous epithelium to grow to full maturity. Deficit or even absence of glycogen can be readily verified by means of *Schiller's* iodine test. The young epithelium appears iodine-bright or iodine-negative. Yet, the process of differentiation finally does take place, in the course of time, and so only the margin of squamous epithelium appears iodine-bright in older transformation areas.

With the colourful variety of patterns, it is somewhat difficult to describe the colposcopic image obtainable from the transformation zone. The following phases of transformation may be found quite often in coexistence and in colourful mixture:

- Usually distinct but irregularly drawn boundaries between squamous and columnar epithelia, with certain tongues and spits of squamous epithelium advancing and islands of metaplastic squamous epithelium being scattered;
- Islands of columnar epithelium surrounded by finely structured networks of squamous epithelium spits, giving the impression of field reversal;
- Squamous epithelium with numerous „glandular" openings from which clear mucus is discharged in pulsating manner, such pulsating discharge being detectable primarily in responce to acetic acid;
- Ruptured glands with lacerated edges, moderate bleeding, epithelial defects, and grotesque openings;

- Naboth's ovules with clearly visible vessels in often very thin and transparent membranes stretching underneath squamous epithelium and showing regular ramification of vessels; Naboth's ovules may be very large, in certain cases, so that the entire portio may be deformed and the os uteri atypically displaced;
- Whitish areas of pinhead size which may appear as field patterns to the less attentive examiner, but in reality they are cones of squamous epithelium which have grown into preformed crypts of connective tissue and into „glandular" openings.

In summarising the above observations, the point can be made that in the young, open transformation zone the columnar epithelium on the surface of the portio had been replaced, while the „glandular" outlet ducts still are open. Hence, the portio is found to be covered with pale-pink squamous epithelium which has positioned in it an irregular arrangement of pinhead-size holes of open „glands" from which clear, viscous mucus may be discharged in eruptive cycles. The squamous epithelium is irregularly tinted, and vascular patterns are not clearly shaped yet. The epithelium is vulnerable and often impaired by inflammatory infiltrations. Iodine-bright to iodine-negative findings are obtainable from *Schiller*'s iodine test. Membranisation of the old, closed transformation zone has been widely completed. The „glandular" openings are closed. Numerous epithelial swellings of whitish shade are visible, instead of „glands". Also recordable are retention cysts of varying sizes with typically ramified vessels. Regions of differentiated whitish coloration appear in response to acetic acid, and all variants, from iodine-positive to iodine-negative, are recordable by means of *Schiller's* iodine test. As soon as no cysts are any longer detectable, the definition will be secondary original portio, and its epithelium, in many cases, can still be delimited from original epithelium, if acetic acid is applied. Adhesion of this squamous epithelium of the transformation zone to connective tissue stroma of columnar epithelium was found to be closer than hat of the original portio. Squamous epithelium of the closed transformation zone adheres tightly, on account of both its growing into the glands and the formation of cones. Intra-epithelial papillae also have grown from connective tissue into this epithelium. The vascular pattern of the transformation zone is highly variable and difficult to describe. The typical vessels of the transformation zone, located in the stroma and underneath the columnar epithelium, are more or less visible, depending on epithelium thickness. They are usually directed toward the external os uteri, and they are ramified with regularity and continuously declining diameter. The arrangement of those vessels can be concentric or radial relative to the open glands, islands of squamous epithelium, and retention cysts. Intervascular spacings are quite variable, between 0.04 mm and 0.2 mm. While network capillaries are recordable from some areas and hairpin capillaries from others, vascular ramification remains to be the most common form. They are actually arborised, fascicular, varicose or like broom twigs. Variation in calibre does occur, caused by rhythmic narrowing and dilatation. There are also vessels of somewhat cork-screw similarity but with completely normal ramification. Young transformation zones usually are strongly vascularised. Assessment, sometimes, is rendered quite difficult, on account of accompanying inflammation.

The highly vascularised transformation zone remains to be identifiable through all phases of "healing". It is conspicuous for a great number of vessels of relatively large calibres which actually shoot into the transformation zone. Orientation of vessel growth to the external os uteri as well as arborisation and tapered diameter of vessels are the major criteria for assessment. The vessels often can be visualised quite clearly by means of acetic acid which causes fading of epithelium. *Schiller's* iodine test will fail to yield an unambiguous result.

The transformation zone, in conclusion, is the most important area, adjacent to the portio. Processes of malignancy tend to start in that zone in more than 90 per cent of all cases. Metaplasia together with transformation form the basis on which the switch is shifted either towards the development of normal regenerative epithelium or to stepwise canceration. It is the connective tissue stroma of columnar epithelium where rise is given to the growth of normal squamous epithelium or of dysplastic epithelium or of ordinary carcinoma.

4. Inflammatory, infectious, and parasitic lesions to the cervix uteri

Fluor is a specific feature of gynaecological inflammation. Colposcopy, therefore, can make a substantive contribution to the detection and diagnosis of inflammatory processes. The epithelia of vagina and portio are comparable to all other epithelia, in that they have two basically different responses, either partial to total desquamation to ulceration or hyperplastic growth.

The majority of inflammations is not limited to one type of epithelium, but both squamous and columnar epithelia tend to be equally affected.

The following colposcopic findings are recordable from cases of inflammation with epithelial desquamation but without ulceration: The portio is covered with leucorrhoeal fluor of liquid and foamy consistence, similar to trichomoniasis and coccal infections. Fluor resulting from mycosis usually is crumbly and clotted.

In such cases, cleaning will be the only effect of acetic acid. Columnar and squamous epithelia will produce one and the same capillary reaction, in that the superficial vessels appear to be expanded as thick red spots. The colour difference between columnar and squamous epithelia may have disappeared. Exudation from the apex of the vascular axis is a typical phenomenon.

Schiller's iodine test may be an indicator to severity of a given inflammation. The more superficial cellular layers have undergone desquamation, the greater will be the extent to which the area grows iodine-negative. Patterns often seem to be similar to a leopard skin, yellow dots on brown ground. The area can be iodine-negative in the presence of a highly severe inflammation, since no glycogen has yet been stored in deeper cell layers. Successful treatment of the inflammation will restore the epithelial structure to normal condition, whereas vascular criteria of inflammation will continue to be detectable for some time.

The following colposcopic findings proved to be recordable from inflammation with ulceration: The surface of the portio can be covered completely or partially with grey pseudomembranes, with the latters' detachment causing focal haemorrhage. Ulceration proper is characterised by the pattern of erosio vera. Less affected areas come very close to inflammation without ulceration, the pattern described above. Terminal conditions of inflammatory processes may yield the following colposcopic findings. Scleroses are present as residues of inflammations. They develop due to regression of those vessels which, at the beginning, had supplied blood to fresh connective tissue in the process of formation. Scarcely vascularised connective tissue, under these conditions, is pink-grey or grey, depending on the duration of the sclerosis. The grey zone tends to persist, following the use of acetic acid, depending on structure and thickness of covering epithelium, but it will vanish, following *Schiller's* iodine test.

Epithelium which covers a sclerotic area often may be found to be of low quality and fragile and, consequently, highly vulnerable. Stricture and stenosis of the external os uteri may result from recurrent inflammation (including cervix rupture due to curretage and childbirth). A typical special form of sclerotisation was found to occur as a side-effect of locally delimited radiotherapy.

Superficially located teleangiectatic fragile vessels often are observed in sclerotic regions, and problems of adequate interpretation may then be facing the unexperienced user of colposcopy.

Hyperplasia of epithelium is another response to inflammation and may cause epithelium concerned to swell twice to three times of its original dimensions. Proliferation of conjunctive-vascular axes in case of papilloma is an extreme condition, in that context. The following colposcopic findings are recordable from hyperplasia in response to inflammation: Raised or verrucously warped patches develop with obtuse demarcation and begin to stand out even more clearly and distinctively, following application of acetic acid. *Schiller's* iodine test will produce irregularly stained areas. They are iodine-bright, and the less vigilant examiner might confuse them with leucoplakia (keratosis), though the latter is of white brilliancy and iodine-negative.

Colpitis vetularum is a special form of colpitis from which the following colposcopic findings may be obtained: The portio is of pale pink shade and reflective. Turbid, maloderous, and highly liquid secretion usually may be found in the vagina. Shining through very thin epithelium are many network capillaries and also soft, regularly distributed vessels in a plaque which are centripedally oriented to a lymphoid follicle. Iodine-bright to iodine-negative epithelium will be shown as a result of *Schiller's* iodine test.

Colpitis, occurring frequently in pregnant women and in women on oral hormonal contraceptives, is usually of focal manifestation, its appearance being dark-red on account of concomitant lividity. Emphysematous colpitis is a special form, resulting in the development of gas-filled cysts in epithelia of the portio and vagina.

Increased vascularisation of superficial epithelium of the cervix is a typical indicator to an inflammatory process. Hairpin capillaries, sometimes, extend as high as into the stromatic papillae and have two or even three crests (trichomoniasis) at the top of the vascular arch. These vessels, called double capillaries, are described as being comparable with forks, antlers or cloverleaf forms. Direct visual inspection of the vascular arches will render the picture similar to the microscopic image of diplococci, with capillary loops appearing as red stiplets in regular side-by-side arrangement. Severe inflammatory reaction tends to be followed by reduction in intercapillary distance, due to both enlargement of the individual capillaries and an increasing number of functional terminal vessels (*Johannisson, Kolstad, Söderberg*). *Zinser* and *Rosenbauer* have interpreted that very pattern of papillary vessels as a physiological variant of terminal vessels beneath orginal epithelium.

A vascular pattern of particular complexity is recordable from inflammation of the transformation zone. The presence of hyperaemia adds greatly to the fascinating nature of the colposcopic image which is, anyway, highly variegated with ramification, network, and hairpin vessels. Fresh capillaries tend to shoot from original capillaries, and additional capillaries grow from afferent vessels into the inflammatory area (*Kos, Lane*).

This vascular pattern, typically, appears diffused and without distinct delimitation from its environment. The oedematous epithelium is excessively reddened by vascular reaction. The unexperienced examiner may have some problems in interpreting such inflammation-based vascular proliferation, since the pathological vascular pattern is difficult to differentiate from the hairpin type. The author's own experience is likely to suggest that the initial phases of circulatory response are, for all practical purposes, identical with carcinogenesis and inflammation. Processes rather differ from one another, in that benign inflammation is accompanied by reaction of the entire capillary network, whereas with stepwise canceration distinctly outlined and demarcated areas are affected. *Koller* and *Kolstad* found that stepwise canceration was accompanied by enlargement of intercapillary distance.

Differentiation between acute and chronic colpitis will be based on quantity and condition of fluor. High purulence of fluor may be an indicator to acute inflammation. Conspicuous colposcopic findings have been recorded, for example, from one specific inflammation, that is gonorrhoea in childhood and senile age. In patients of these two age groups, gonococci obviously are capable of penetrating epithelium and cause micro-abscesses in it. Similar pictures, which sometimes turned into bizarre tumorous or verrucous structures, have been recorded also from pregnant women. Such apparently atypical vascular developments, in concomitance with proliferations, often have led to suspicion of carcinoma of the cervix in gravidity.

Tuberculosis has been one of the very rare findings recordable from the portio. It has caused the development of flattened, apparently punched out ulcerations with sharp edges and considerable inclination to bleeding which could occur simultaneously on a number of sites. Luetic primary sore has been found to occur rarely on the portio. It is characterised by solitary occurrence and may be very similar in appearance to tuberculous ulcer. Differential diagnosis is relatively easy by taking a swab of irritative secretion.

Erosio vera means nothing but loss of epithelial coat. It is usually of traumatic, iatrogenic or inflammatory origin but rarely caused by carcinoma. The exposed region from which epithelium has been lost is colposcopically represented as a dark-red area which contrasts clearly from its surrounding. Fragments of torn-off epithelial coat may often be detectable at marginal points. The acetic acid test has proved to be an effective tool for safe differentiation between pseudo-erosion and ectopy. Erosio vera is not accompanied by white discoloration of columnar epithelium. No reaction is produced in erosio vera by connective tissue stroma. Treatment for inflammation has to be followed by highly scrupulous follow-up checking, since erosio vera may be of carcinomatous genesis. The following aspects should be given particular attention by the colposcopic examiner:

- Assessment of marginal areas of erosio vera, with particular consideration to be given to the vascular configuration;
- Assessment of the extent to which erosio vera stands out from its environment;
- Assessment of surface and structure of erosio vera;
- Assessment of colour and consistency of erosio vera bottom.

Non-carcinomatous erosio vera will not exhibit any atypical changes in the area by which it is surrounded, such as floor (punctuation), field pattern (mosaic) or leucoplakia (keratosis). It will be situated flush with the epithelium, its surface being regular and even. It will be of diffusedly red coloration, with no detectable yellowish or glassy regions. The vascular pattern is that of normal connective tissue and bears no atypical signs. This form of erosio vera is transient and properly responsive to therapy.

Carcinomatous erosio vera, however, will colposcopically show in its environment conspicuous epithelial regions, such as floor or punctuation, field pattern or mosaic, leucoplakia or keratosis, as well as atypical vessels. Its surface is situated clearly beneath the level of its environment and, quite often, comparable with a mountain landscape. It is of yellowish colour or has at least strongly yellowish foci. Atypical vessels of different shapes are recordable from stroma. Even the slightest suspicion should be settled immediately by histological examination.

5. Suspicious colposcopic findings – atypical transformation zone

5.1. Atypical transformation (by delimited definition)

(Actypical transformation zone, according to *Glatthaar*, abnormal transformation zone, according to *Hinselmann*, uncommon transformation zone, according to *Mestwerdt*, *Wespi*, suspicious transformation zone, according to *Ganse*)

A multiplicity of pathological findings has been summarised under the cover term of atypical transformation zone and its synonyms. Those findings, quite often, are overlooked, since they are not strikingly conspicuous by expansion and pronunciation. The term has been, likewisely, applied to findings which cannot be associated with *Hinselmann's* classical "matrix" regions.

Highly differentiated findings have been quoted and proposed by different authors as criteria of the atypical transformation zone. *Glatthaar*, for example, has stressed extensive vascularisation with atypical vessels patterns and poor transparency of epithelium of opaque, grey-whitish to yellowish coloration.

Burkhardt has emphasised the importance of washed out shade, negative response to iodine, and distinct demarcation from normal epithelium.

Vinegar-white epithelium, areas of field patterns, papillary formation with corkscrew capillaries, hornifield or whitish "glandular openings", differentiation in level, as well as iodine-brightness to iodine-negativity are considered suspicious criteria by *Ganse* and *Holtorff*. Quite a problem has been posed, in that context, by the need for differentiation of inflammatory processes with various forms of epithelial proliferation and for interpretation of various forms of vascularisation. Colour deviation may result also from inflammation caused by tissue oedema and microcellular infiltration.

An atypical transformation zone, quite obviously, differs from a normal transformation zone, in that faulty differentiation appears to have taken place primarily, in the process of metaplastic regeneration, and to have continued to the extent of definite transformation.

An atypical transformation zone may be colposcopically characterised by small classical "matrix" regions, usually overlooked at the beginning, conspicuous strengthening of vascular contours, and changes in the vascular pattern, such as variation in calibres, adaptative vascular hypertrophy, corkscrew capillaries, hairpin vessels, and numerous elongated thin-calibre vessels, often in parallel and with no ramification.

Also involved are epithelial defects, differences in level with mound-like boundaries and papillary formation, hornified and white-rimmed "glandular openings", as well as grey-white discoloration of epithelium following application of acetic acid.

The atypical transformation zone has been subdivided into three degrees by *Coppleson*, *Pixley*, and *Reid*:

1. Shallow white epithelium, with or without fine-calibre vessels;
2. Shallow white epithelium, with or without large-calibre, irregular vessels;
3. Very white epithelium with large-calibre and glomerular vessels, irregular surface topography, and papillary epithelium.

Hk. Bauer found the following criteria to be important to an atypical transformation zone:

- Vinegar-white epithelium which differs form leucoplakia (keratosis), in that it turns white only under the impact of acetic acid;
- Open "glands" with red base in vinegar-white epithelium, often with whitish hornification rim, but also with red rim, pitted or with papillary projections comparable to glove fingers;
- Minor erosions, mosaic, punctuation, leucoplakia (keratosis);
- All forms of vascular abnormality, including hairpin and cork-screw capillaries, variation in calibres, bizarre and torn vessels;
- Differences in level.

He also felt that larger areas of punctuation should be associated with such findings, and so should mosaic and leucoplakia (keratosis), however, without defining those cases as atypical transformation zone.

The author feels, after all, that emphasis should be laid on detectability and diagnosis of atypical vascular ramification. Atypically ramified vessels have already been described by *Hinselmann* and, more recently, by *Kirsch* and *Rieck*. Such vessels are somewhat strange mainly for their rigidity, monotony, and visual regularity.

5.2. Leucoplakia (keratosis)

Leucoplakia, the white spot, has been the first classical "matrix" region postulated by *Hinselmann*. It had been macroscopically detected even earlier by *von Franque*, *Hinselmann's* teacher, and described by him as precancerosis. Its proper interpretation has continued to prove difficult even in colposcopic diagnosis in our days. Leucoplakia may include not only benign proliferative processes, but also manifestations of precursor phases or early forms of carcinoma of the cervix. Adequate judgement of leucoplakia (keratosis) for its malignant or benign potentials was found to depend strongly on location, appearance, condition, and delimitation from surrounding tissue. Most various findings have been summarised under the cover term of leucoplakia (keratosis). There may be solitary or multiply distributed white stains, similar to patches of oil-paint, which may cover parts of the portio and extend to the vaginal fornix. Leucoplakia always is raised above the level of surrounding mucous membrane and consists of epithelial layers of parakeratosis and hyperkeratosis which are of reduced transparency on account of three factors, high protein level, layer thickness, and nuclear density. No staining will occur in response to *Schiller's* iodine test due to complete absence of intra-epithelial glycogen. Appearance usually is not changed either by acetic acid. Many types of leucoplakia (keratosis) are easily detachable and vulnerable, and so the colposcopic image is likely to undergo substantive change within few days. The vascular pattern of leucoplakia (keratosis) cannot be judged until the layers of parakeratosis and hyperkeratosis have been removed, since transparency is poor, as mentioned above. Atypical vessels of the hairpin type are often recordable. *Hinselmann* defined those findings as floor of leucoplakia. Structures of field pattern (mosaic), sometimes, are detectable, in the context of leucoplakia (keratosis). A variety of patterns is actually recordable from leucoplakia areas by histological testing, from benign hypertrophic abnormal epithelium through different stages of epithelial dysplasia to ordinary carcinoma. The potential error implied in assessment of leucoplakia (keratosis) by means of colposcopy is even greater than that implied in cytological examination. Leucoplakia (keratosis) is colposcopically recordable from something between one and four per cent of patients. Attempts have been made to define various forms of leucoplakia (keratosis), with the view to providing information about an index of malignancy.

5.2.1. Tender leucoplakia (keratosis)

A very thin and tender stratification of hyperkeratotic cells is built up on the portio, primarily in young patients. Tender leucoplakia may persist for years, with no malignant potential, and should be considered as inflammatory proliferation. Leucoplakia (keratosis) may occur also in conjunction with vaginal and uterine prolapse as a reflection of adaptation of epithelium to environmental change. This is not assumed either to be a risk of malignancy.

5.2.2. Simple leucoplakia (keratosis)

This is one of the relatively frequent findings, with solitary or multiple occurrence, which, in many cases, can be wiped off easily. Colposcopically visualised is the floor (punctuation) or field pattern (mosaic). There usually are several stages of dysplasia.

5.2.3. Squamous leucoplakia (keratosis)

The colposcopic impression is that of a fissured or ruptured horny surface, quite often with some sort of coarse field pattern. It often is an indicator to carcinomatous alteration and, therefore, should be histologically elucidated, with no delay. Its combination with field pattern (mosaic) and floor (punctuation) is quite common. Marginal leucoplakic coating of ordinary carcinoma is a special form of leucoplakia.

5.2.4. Tough leucoplakia (keratosis)

The term of tough leucoplakia has been used by various authors, generally, to define squamous leucoplakia. Tough leucoplakia stands out from its surroundings in verrucous or papillary shape. Carcinoma is a frequent result of histological examination, particularly in cases of increased haemorrhagic tendency.

Tender and simple leucoplakias are likely to undergo regression to a great extent, over the years. While leucoplakia, certainly, is not necessarily a condition of precancerosis, it is a good reason for careful follow-up and thorough diagnosis.

5.3. Floor (punctuation)

According to *Hinselmann*, the floor of leucoplakia, or briefly "floor", has been defined as an area of atypical epithelium which has been deprived of its leucoplakic cover shield. Yet, today, it has been generally accepted that the image of floor can be colposcopically recorded also in the absence of leucoplakia.
Hinselmann and others found the floor, as the basis of leucoplakia, characterised by clearly projecting papillary vessels, yellowish to pink discoloration in contrast to surrounding tissue, distinct delimitation of the area affected, usually below the surrounding level, whitish discoloration following application of acetic acid, and negative response to *Schiller's* iodine test.

Glatthaar emphasised, in particular, the following criteria: moderately lowered floor surface with clearly visible red spots of superficially situated capillary loops of connective tissue which tended to start bleeding moderately, on contact, all on yellowish coloration.

Cramer described the floor as a white to yellowish discolorated region with some red stippling caused by capillary loops. Today, there are many authors (*Ganse, Mestwerdt, Wespi, Zinser, Coupez, Kolstad, Limburg, Koller, Kos, Coppleson, Hk. Bauer, Stafl*) by whom the colposcopic image of the floor (punctuation) is considered the product of an atypical metaplasia of ectopic columnar epithelium in which all folds and indentations of the transformation zone are filled up with metaplastic, atypical squamous epithelium, with only the papillae of the former ectopy "surviving". Increasing epithelial proliferation, accompanied by papillary compression, is followed by dilatation of vessels and their proliferation to the surface. Intercapillary distance is likely to grow in the process of advancing carcinogenesis, quite different from inflammation. Hence, today, the definition of floor (punctuation) has to be conceived as a cover term for all findings which are similar to what has been described first by *Hinselmann,* without being a nosological unit. Colposcopic findings of floor may be classified as follows, depending on the degree of atypia:

5.3.1. Tender floor (punctuation)

Tender floor, usually, does not grow manifest until acetic acid is applied. No-glycogen, still immature metaplastic epithelium without malignant potential forms the histological substrate. Depicted by colposcopy is a plane surface which turns whitish, when swabbed with acetic acid of three per cent concentration. It is distinctly demarcated from its surrouding area but flush with the latter. The area concerned will produce negative response to *Schiller's* iodine test. The capillary arches of the papillary vessels tend to flash as red spots in regular intervals, when exposed to incident light. Hence, their naming of punctuation. *Hk. Bauer* found this picture to be recordable quite frequently from young women with ovarian insufficiency or women on contraceptives or patients in the menopause.

5.3.2. Simple floor (punctuation)

Colposcopically, the regions concerned are distinctly delimited from their environment. They may be flush or lowered, with whitish and yellowish coloration or reddish. Red spots are visible on the capillary arches, sometimes, irregularly spaced. The epithelium is likely to undergo some paling, when exposed to acetic acid. No change occurs to the capillary arches. This form of floor, too, produces clearly negative response to iodine.

5.3.3. Papillary floor (punctuation)

This is the colposcopic representation of severely changed pathological epithelium, including carcinoma. The areas of papillary floor usually are distinctly demarcated from their surroundings. Raised papillae, like verrucous nodes, are recordable from such demarcated areas. The papillary vessels appear to be nodular, and intercapillary spacings quite clearly are larger and irregular. The papillary floor is of glassy, yellowish colour and turns more to white in response to acetic acid. The vessels proper were not found to respond to acetic acid. This severely atypical epithelium has, most conspicuously, exhibited washed out iodine brightness in response to *Schiller's* iodine test. "Fingerlike processes", as described by *Cullen,* are detectable from certain forms of floor. The vessels, of cork-screw winding and located in uneven ground, often are bizarre in shape and intertwined. Occasionally, there may be hairpin capillaries which run in parallel with the surface. Secondary cork-screw capillaries, so to say, originate from their apical arches.

Floor was found to differ from the regular pattern of inflammation, with alterations all over the place, in that the following typical characteristics proved to be recordable from it:

- Change in colour, with dark-red discoloration of inflammatory foci being substituted by pink, yellow, and white;
- Colour is further changed to white in response to acetic acid;
- A distinctly delimited iodine-negative to iodine-bright region is likely to develop in response to *Schiller's* iodine test;
- Areas affected may be plane, embedded below surrounding level or polypously raised, depending on severity of the pathological process;
- Most various phases in the formation of capillary loops my be observed, depending on floor atypia, with normal vessels, varicosity in descending vessels, baskets, clubs, and glomeruloid capillary loops being jammed in narrow space. There may be hairpin or cork-screw capillaries in other regions, with secondary loops of vessels developing from them.
- Additional pathological findings often are recordable by colposcopy, within one

given area or side by side, but distinctly delimited from normal tissue, for example, various forms of leucoplakia (keratosis) and field pattern (mosaic).

5.3.4. Stippled floor (punctuation)

While the presence of papillary floor usually marks a transitional phase towards carcinomatous exophyte, stippled floor, according to *Hinselmann*, clearly is carcinoma. His definition of stippled floor has been, as follows: "These are small-field changes within a distinct region, and one wonders, if it should be defined as field pattern (mosaic) or floor. Those small fields are of yellowish shade and similar to nests of wild-growing epithelium."

5.4. Field pattern (mosaic)

Hinselmann considered the field pattern (mosaic) the third classical matrix region. He felt that field pattern was closely associated with leucoplakia (keratosis). In his description of the colposcopic image of field pattern, he referred to areas of yellowish-white small polygonal fields which consisted of blocks of atypical epithelium and were somewhat in a relationship with the "glands" of the transformation zone. Those fields, without vessels themselves, were surrounded by densely packed vessel-containing stromatic papillae which, histologically, were infiltrated with microcells and coated with thin epithelium.

He also saw those colposcopic images where each of the fields showed in its centre "glandular" openings with whitish to yellowish frames.

The field pattern could be more clearly delimited from normal epithelium, following application of three-per-cent acetic acid. Fields turned more to white, giving more contrast to the red spots and vascular lines in their own frames. Field pattern areas produced clearly negative reactions to *Schiller's* iodine test.

The colposcopic image of field pattern was thought already by *Hinselmann* to have originated from subcolumnar epithelial cells of ectopic mucous membrane through indirect metaplasia. He also thought that the "glands" were first lost in the development of that field pattern, on account of block formation of atypical epithelium. *Kolstad* and *Stafl* found themselves in agreement with those views, and they, too, considered field pattern a product of atypical metaplasia, with various phases being undergone. The first phase, as they proposed, was one with extremely strong inclination to regression, field reversal. That phase is rarely observed, on account of its high speed and thus short duration, and it is likely to result from growth pressure of atypical epithelium. This finding will be expounded in greater detail. Yet, first, it tends to be followed by phases of steadily mounting growth pressure of atypical epithelial blocks which compress the vessels of the stromatic papillae to the shape of a basket-like network.

Field pattern (mosaic) stands for a large variety of different findings so far described and defined by most various examiners. All of them have the following criteria in common:

- Presence of round, quadratic, rhombic, oblong, bizarre large or small fields, one monotonous unit or a compound picture;
- Areas of atypical epithelium are delimited by connective tissue septa in which once regularly arranged vessels are now compressed; compressed vessels may be positioned perpendicularly or in parallel to surface and exhibit pathological alterations in shape and diameter;
- Fields are rendered more to the white, and colposcopic pictures will become clearer by three-per-cent acetic acid;
- All field pattern areas produce negative reaction to *Schiller's* iodine test, with iodine-brightness being a rare exception.

The vascular structure of field pattern can be highly variegated. There may be fine, trichoid or relatively tough and dilated vessels arranged regularly or irregularly in connective tissue. Intercapillary spacing is a major indicator to epithelial atypia. Growing intercapillary spacings, caused by disappearance of stromatic papillae, suggest aggravating severity of the pathological condition of the epithelium concerned. "Field pattern vessels" may be rows of hairpin capillaries, in irregular directions or parallel with the surface. Also recorded were mutually anastomising vessels, often elevated to a level very close beneath the thinned epithelial surface. Angiographic findings have suggested that vessels which, colposcopically, appeared as straight lines actually were of corrugated shape due to partial ectasia of vascular walls. The following description of various forms of field pattern has been compiled in an order to describe the severity of epithelial atypia.

5.4.1. Field reversal (mosaic)

Field reversal has already been mentioned as being one of the relatively rare findings which is only conditionally a phenomenon that should come under the heading of "field pattern". Several authors have interpreted and defined field reversal as the colposcopically detectable expression of atypical metaplastic transformation in an initial phase. This phase, probably, is characterised by very intensive blood supply. Its response to three-per-cent acetic acid differs from that of genuine field pattern by emergence of polygonal to circular reddish fields, caused by stromatic papillae which are vaulting towards the surface.

Such "reversed fields" are delimited by white strands of avascular metaplastic epithelium. This colposcopic picture has been recordable from pregnant women or girls in puberty.

5.4.2. Tender field pattern (mosaic)

The colposcopic picture of tender field pattern is a safe indicator to merely moderate atypia. It has been recorded most often from large portio regions in very young women and women with ovarian insufficiency and, more recently, in growing numbers of patients on hormonal contraceptives. Colposcopically visible are tender, small, fairly uniform round or rhombic fields which are delimited by red vascular lines. They are hardly visible at all, if no acetic acid is used. Those findings may persist throughout years, but they tend to disappear very soon, once the hormonal situation is getting normalised.

5.4.3. Simple field pattern (mosaic)

Fields are located at the very level of the mucous membrane. They are clearly identifiable and usually of regular shape. Vessels are delimited by composed and regular lines, with no significant enlargement of intercapillary spacings. No particularly conspicuous vascular atypia is recordable. Slight to moderate dysplasia may be one of the more frequent histological findings.

5.4.4. Raised field pattern (mosaic)

Colposcopically, atypical epithelium is irregularly raised above the level of normal mucous membrane, which is one of the immediate impressions, right at the first glance. Administration of acetic acid then seems to change those fields more to the white and to make them swelling. Fields are avascular and of glassy, washed out appearance.

5.4.5. Keratinised, raised field pattern (mosaic)

Keratinised and raised field pattern was found to differ from simply raised field pattern by, occasionally, excessive occurrence of parakeratotic superimposed deposits which stand out clearly from the surface. This finding may be so strongly pronounced that it can be hardly differentiated from squamous leucoplakia (keratosis). The histological substrate usually is carcinoma in situ or early-invasive carcinoma.

5.4.6. Funnel field pattern (mosaic)

This extremely rare finding, described by *Hinselmann*, is mentioned for the sake of completeness. It might be interpreted, just as well, as a variant of keratinised, raised field pattern. Colposcopically visible is a small horny cone on top of each raised field, similar in appearance to a small cap or funnel.

5.4.7. Yellow raised field pattern (mosaic)

Raised fields of clearly yellowish colour stand out irregularly from the surface of surrounding epithelium. Blurred or fading outlines, glassy field appearance, and occasional iodine-brightness are urgent colposcopic indicators to the presence of carcinoma.

5.4.8. Bizarre field pattern (mosaic)

The name of bizarre field pattern has been coined with reference to the frequently bizarre forms and sizes of the fields involved which may overlap and flow into one another. Raised fields may coexist with somewhat keratinising areas. The vascular scene may be a highly variable and colourful picture. There may be dilated vessels with various orientations. Bizarre field pattern often is a finding complementary to ordinary carcinomatous ulceration or exophyte.

5.4.9. Trough field pattern (mosaic)

This phenomenon was found to differ from all the above field patterns, in that the pathologically affected epithelium is actually expanded vertically downward into larger depths. The fields, consequently, come to lie beneath the epithelial surface of surrounding normal epithelium. "Glandular" openings were found to be embedded in the troughs. Vessels are not particularly conspicuous or suspicious. This colposcopic finding should be treated with greatest caution, since the direction of epithelial growth may have been caused by an infiltratingly growing carcinoma, without any warning signal being given by the vessels.

5.5. Combined forms of leucoplakia, floor, and field pattern (keratosis, punctuation, and mosaic)

While the occurrence of combined forms has been associated to the category of atypical transformation zone by certain examiners, the very combination of "matrix" regions is being considered by other hard evidence to the presence of severe pathological changes.

Such colposcopic findings should be carefully followed up cytologically and histologically. Since a description has been given in greater detail of individual and separate occurrences of leucoplakia, floor, and field pattern, no explanation will be necessary of their combinational manifestations. Besides, it would be quite impossible to give even an approximate verbal account of the colourful variety of those combinations.

6. Erosia vera

Erosio vera is defined as an epithelial defect in a circumscribed region of the portio cervicis uteri. The colposcopic image is unambiguous. The region is of diffused red to dark-red, with no reflection of incident light being detectable. Colour does not change in response to acetic acid due to the absence od reactive epithelium. Displayed in the region of erosio vera are spots of diffused haemorrhage, getting worse by contact with the vulnerable connective tissue. It is absolutely necessary to elucidate the genesis of erosio vera. The following criteria may be helpful in differentiating carcinoma from artefact or mechanical insult:

- Level of erosio vera relative to surroundings;
- Surface relief of the erosion proper;
- Colour;
- Vascular pattern in erosio vera;
- Condition of marginal regions of erosio vera and blood flow to the vessels of those marginal regions.

With non-carcinomatous erosio vera, the level of the defect is almost identical with the level of the mucous membrane. The surface of the erosion proper is plane and with no indentations. The uniformly red coloration, sometimes, may have been disrupted by haemorrhagic, fibrinous superimposed deposits or by regularly arranged yellowish shining lymph follicles. This should be interpreted as a sign of long persistance of the erosion, but it may cause problems of diagnosis. The vascular pattern of the exposed connective tissue stroma is as unconspicuous as that described in the context of original portio. Vessel coloration may appear to be strengthened for absence of epithelial coat. Tilted or ruptured layers of epithelium, often, may be recorded from the marginal regions of non-carcinomatous erosio vera. The margin does not exhibit any bulging or undermining. Non-carcinomatous erosio vera will respond to adequate treatment by rapid healing, with no residual defect being left.

Carcinomatous erosio vera, on the other hand, tends to exhibit the first conspicuous changes even on inspection of the level of surrounding intact tissue. The level of carcinomatous erosio vera is ulceratively lowered or raised exophytically above the surrounding intact mucous membrane. Both findings also may be recordable in coexistence. Hence, the surface of this erosion is comparable to a range of mountains. Colposcopically, the tissue gives the impression of very poor tenacity and high brittleness, with its yellowish coloration changing in intensity. Atypical vessels, occurring in highly variable forms, actually back up suspicion of carcinoma.

The margin of carcinomatous erosio vera often appears to be raised. Sometimes, it may be pitted and undermined. The surrounding epithelium is altered in terms of classical "matrix regions" or in terms of atypical transformation by delimited definition. Vascular patterns are changed accordingly. Comparatively reliable prediction of carcinoma can be made, in such case, on the basis of colposcopy alone.

7. Carcinoma

The points made so far are likely to suggest quite clearly that the great variety of pathological changes in squamous epithelium of the portio, colposcopically defined as atypical transformation zone, leucoplakia (keratosis), floor (punctuation), and field pattern (mosaic), may conceal both relatively low levels of malignant transformation or complete carcinoma. Three major groups may be established in a bid to order all colposcopic findings which seem to bear relevance in terms of carcinoma.

Colposcopic findings of histological correspondence with carcinoma

1. **Tough forms of "matrix" regions**
1.1. Squamous leucoplakia (keratosis)
1.2. Papillary floor (tough punctuation)
1.3. Raised, raised keratinised, and yellow field pattern (tough mosaic)
1.4. Atypical transformation zone
1.5. Combined forms of 1.1. through 1.3.
2. **Preclinical early forms of carcinoma**
2.1. Preclinical exophytic carcinoma
2.2. Preclinical endophytic carcinoma
2.3. Adenoplastic and anaplastic carcinoma
3. **Ordinary carcinoma**

The first group of colposcopic findings, with their histological substrate being carcinoma, has been described in detail in the previous sections.

Reference will now be made to the second group. Preclinical exophytic carcinoma, listed under 2.1., is characterised by sizeable difference of its own level from the level of surrounding clinically intact mucous membrane. Proper diagnosis is comparatively easy, on account of a number of unmistakable features, such as glassy yellowish-white to yellowish-brown colour, strawberry-like appearance of the surface, caused by yellowish tops of more deeply embedded carcinoma nests, as well as trend to diffuse haemorrhage. The tissue affected gives the impression of being boiled, after having been exposed to acetic acid, three per cent in concentration, and those vessels which are situated on top of the surface are bizarre in shape and variable in calibre. The vascular pattern has, quite generally, become a decisive criterion of assessment. Colposcopic findings recordable from preclinical exophytic carcinoma are highly differentiated and even contradictory, with adaptive vascular hypertrophy, on the one hand, and adaptively sufficient deformative vascular hypertrophy, on the other. The former is characterised by dilated and hypertrophic capillaries, coiled like cork-screws and with steadily enlarging intercapillary spacings, while the latter may show avascular tissue areas and in them bizarre cork-screw capillaries (*Mestwerdt*), hairpin vessels (*Ganse*), and elongated epithelial tubes (*Chiari*). Vessels also are atypically ramified and highly variegated in calibre. The vascular pattern, as a whole, appears to be confused and chaotic. Insufficient deformative vascular hypertrophy then may be seen in the period of transition to ordinary carcinoma.

Preclinical endophytic carcinoma, listed under 2.2., is, in its initial phases, more or less identical with the criteria of carcinomatous erosio vera. It is likely to occur in regions without invasive growth as a red surface from which all epithelium has been removed, its topography again being comparable to a mountain landscape. Again, particular reference should be made to the presence of small yellowish washed out nests of round or angular shapes, that is more deeply situated carcinoma epithelium. Those nests actually determine the direction of infiltrative growth of endophytic carcinoma. Advancing carcinoma growth is accompanied by deeper penetration of the carcinomatous ulcer, and carcinoma sequesters will detach due to poor supply of the tumorous tissue. Deep vascular plexus then are exposed to bring in focus disarrayed large-calibre vessels, some of them being frightfully thick and filled to bursting point or even thrombotic. Inflammatory infiltration often may be recorded from the marginal area of carcinomatous ulcer which may have attached to it radially arranged hairpin-like vessels or other vessels, as described under 1.1. through 1.3. The colour of the carcinoma tissue is likely to change from areas with dark-red blood flow underneath to typical glassy yellowish carcinoma tissue and white friable necroses.

Preclinical adenocarcinoma and anaplastic carcinoma, listed under 2.3., are likely to present certain colposcopic peculiarities which may prove deceptive to the unexperienced examiner. Plenty of fine parallel capillaries, with no ramification at all, is a typical vascular feature both early carcinomas have in common. They are all arranged very close to one another, their intercapillary spacings being normal.

The explanation offered for that deviating vascular pattern by *Kolstad* and *Stafl* is the origin of those atypical vessels from central capillary network of columnar epithelial papillae. Hence, those carcinomas must be supplied from a centralised capillary system. Squamous cell carcinomas, on the other hand, are supplied from peripheral vessels which encircle epithelial blocks without penetrating them. Both the endophytic and exophytic forms of ordinary carcinoma, listed under 3, are detectable even without colposcopy. Vascular patterns on friable, easily tearable, whitish to yellowish washed out epithelium are clearly pronounced and, therefore, unambiguous even to the unexperienced examiner. Immensely elongated and expanded hairpin capillaries have next to them glomerulated vessels of changing diameters. Numerous varicose vessels with vascular ruptures are situated, in undisrupted continuity, in the very same plane. Thrombosis and underside haemorrhage are additional phenomena. Vessels may be dilated but in uniform pattern, with the network type of ordinary carcinoma, according to *Koller*, *Kolstad*, and *Johannisson*. Avascular and necrotic areas as well as atypical ramification vessels, in particular, mean hard evidence to the presence of carcinoma. Thin-calibre vessels, directionally oriented to the sites of tumour growth and with intercapillary spacings in excess of 450 μm, often are recordable from marginal regions.

8. Vascular criteria of transformational stages in cervix uteri (Johannisson, Kolstad, Söderberg)

8.1. Dysplasias

— Tender, unconspicuous irregular floor formations with smooth surface, moderately dilated vessels of the hairpin type, some of them elongated and curled; moderate enlargement of intercapillary spacings;

— Tender, simple, unconspicuous, and irregular formations of field patterns with smooth surface; hairpin vessels arranged in rows, as described also in the context of floor formations; fine, dilated terminal vessels parallel to surface; moderate enlargement of intercapillary spacings.

8.2. Carcinoma in situ

— Conspicuously tough irregular floor formations with papillary surface; strongly dilated hairpin-type vessels with top of vascular arch nest-shaped or glomerulated or strongly elongated in parallel with surface and coiled; intercapillary spacings clearly enlarged;

— Conspicuously tough irregular field pattern formations with blocks raised on surface; hairpin-type vessels or strongly dilated and irregularly curved terminal vessels, forming coarsely interlaced network, orientated in parallel with surface, and arranged in rows; significant enlargement of intercapillary spacings.

8.3. Early invasive carcinoma

Intercapillary spacings are enlarged by factors of two or three, appearance being that of carcinoma in situ but more toughly structured; scattered occurrence of clearly atypical irregular ramification vessels.

8.4. Ordinary carcinoma

Dimensions, calibres, directions, arrangements, ramifications, and intercapillary spacings of extremely atypical carcinomatous vessels are highly irregular, confused, and even chaotic.

8.5. Adenoplastic and anaplastic carcinomas

A countless mass of extremely fine and elongated parallel capillaries with no mutual ramification and normal intercapillary spacings is arranged in high density.

9. References

Almendral, A. C., G. Szalmay, L. Jochum and *H. Müller:* Vor- und Frühstadien des Zervixkarzinoms (Preliminary and Early Phases of Cervical Carcinoma) Fortschr. Med. 92 (1974), 1007–1048

Anderes, E., and *H. J. Wespi:* Der heutige Stand der Früherfassung des Portiokarzinoms mittels der Kolposkopie (Present Position in Early Detection of Portio Carcinoma by means of Colposcopy) Geburtsh. u. Frauenk. 3 (1941), 248

Andrys, J. K., Vacha, M. Rosol and *J. Kopecny:* Präkanzerosen der Cervix uteri in der Schwangerschaft (Precanceroses of Cervix Uteri in Gravidity) Zbl. Gynäkol. 96 (1974), 1012–1015

Antoine, T., and *U. Grünberger:* Atlas der Kolpomikroskopie (Atlas of Colpomicroscopy) Georg Thieme, Stuttgart 1956

Bajardi, F., W. R. Lang, A. de Moraes and *I. P. Rieper:* Kolposkopie der Cervix uteri nach Irradiation (Colposcopic Examination of Cervix Uteri, following Irradiation) Acta cytol. (Chicago) 3 (1960), 369–371

Bargheer, R., and *J. Erbslöh:* Geschwulstartige Gefäßneubildung der Portio (Tumorous Neovasculogenesis of Portio) Z. Geburtsh. Gynäk. 155 (1960)

Beruffi, I., N. Augusto, S. Bighetti and *E. Marcolini:* Betrachtung von über 1000 kolposkopischen Untersuchungen (Account of more than 1,000 Colposcopic Examinations) An bras. Cincc. 56 (1963), 131–136

Bauer, Hk.: Die Sanierung der Portio uteri mit Albothyl als Krebsprophylaxe in der ambulanten Praxis — Dokumentation der Befunde mit Farb-Kolpofotografie (Use of Albothyl for Sanitation of Uterine Portio in Ambulatory Practice — Documentation of Findings with Colour-Colpophotography) Medizinische 10 (1959), 1645–1657

Bauer, Hk.: Langzeitbeobachtungen bei atypischem Epithel — nach einem Vortrag auf dem 5. Weltkongress für Gynäkologie und Geburtshilfe in Sydney 1967 (Long-Term Observation of Atypical Epithelium — from a lecture presented at the 5th World Congress of Gynaecology and Obstetrics in Sydney 1967) Med. Welt 19 (N.F.) (1968), 2048–2050

Bauer, Hk.: Die Bedeutung der Kolposkopie bei der Frühdiagnostik des Kollumkarzinoms in der täglichen Praxis (Relevance of Colposcopy in Every-Day Practice to Early Diagnosis of Cervical Carcinoma) Frauenarzt 11 (1970), 200–202

Bauer, Hk.: Zur Frage einer Vereinfachung der Nomenklatur bei der Kolposkopie (Simplification of Colposcopic Nomenclature) Frauenarzt 13 (1972), 137–138

Bauer, Hk.: Kolposkopie (Colposcopy) Diagnostik 5 (1972), 528–530

Bauer, Hk.: Die Bedeutung der kolpofotografischen Dokumentation bei Langzeitbeobachtungen von dysplastischem Epithel der Cervix uteri — Vortrag auf der 1. Arbeitstagung der Arbeitsgemeinschaft „Cervix uteri" 1972 (Role of Colpophotographic Documentation in Long-Term Observation of Dysplastic Epithelium of Cervix Uteri — Lecture presented at 1st Meeting of "Cervix Uteri" Working Group 1972) Mitteilungsdienst der Gesellschaft zur Bekämpfung der Krebskrankheiten Nordrhein-Westfalen 6 (1973), 939–949

Bauer, Hk.: Kolposkopie (Colposcopy). Arch. Gynäk. 214 (1973), 240–241

Bauer, Hk.: Kolposkopische Kriterien der atypischen Umwandlungszone (Colposcopic Criteria of Atypical Transformation Zone) — Vortrag auf der 3. Arbeitstagung „Cervix uteri" (Lecture at 3rd "Cervix Uteri" Meeting), May 1st to 5th, 1976, Wiesbaden

Bauer, Hk.: Farbatlas der Kolposkopie (Coloured Atlas of Colposcopy). F. K. Schattauer Verlag Stuttgart–New York, 1976

Berger, J. and *H. Wenner-Mangen:* La Colposcopie (Colposcopy) Gynaecologie et Obstetrique 52 (1953), 3, 303–324

Bergleiter, R., and *H. Bettzieche:* Klinische und kolposkopische Befunde bei Präkanzerosen der Cervix uteri — ein Beitrag zur Wertigkeit einer Auswahlzytologie (Clinical and Colposcopic Findings from Precanceroses of Cervix Uteri — Rating of A Selective Cytological Testing Procedure). Zbl. Gynäk. 97 (1975), 12–19

Bergsjo, P., O. Koller and *P. Kolstad:* The vascular pattern of trichomonas vaginalis cervicitis, Acta Cytol. 7 (1963), 292

Beric, B., and H. Smolka: Über den Einfluß der in der Kolposkopie angewandten Reagenzien auf das Zellbild des Portioabstriches (Effects of Reagents, used in Colposcopy, on Cellular Pattern of the Portio Swab). Geburtsh. u. Frauenheilk. 18 (1958), 852–864

Bolten, K. A., and *W. E. Jaques:* Introduction in Colposcopy, Grune & Stratton, New York 1960

Bolten, K. A.: Practical Colposcopy Early Cervical and Vaginal Cancer, Clinical Obstetrics and Gynaeco-

logy, Hoeber Medical Division, New York (1967), 808—837
Boschann, H. W.: Kolposkopie (Colposcopy). Z. ärztl. Fortbild. 52 (1963), 167—170
Brandl, K., and *V. Grünberger:* Der Wert verschiedener Spezialuntersuchungen für die Beurteilung makroskopisch unverdächtiger Erosionen (Usefulness of Various Special Procedures for Examination of Macroscopically Unsuspicious Erosions). Geburtsh. u. Frauenheilk. 14 (1954), 434—450
Bredland, R.: Kolposkopische Diagnose der gynokologischen Trichomoniasis (Colposcopic Diagnosis of Gynaecological Trichomoniasis). Geburtsh. u. Frauenheilk. 25 (1965), 815—821
Bret, J., and *F. Coupez:* Kolposkopie bei normaler und abnormaler Cervix in der Schwangerschaft und post partuus (Colposcopic Inspection of Normal and Abnormal Cervix in Pregnancy and Postpartum). Acta Cytol. 3 (1959), 61—68
Bret, J., and *F. Coupez:* Colposcopie (Colposcopy). Masson & Cie., Paris 1960
Bret, J., and *F. Coupez:* Colposcopie (Colposcopy). Encyclopédie medico-chirurgicale, Paris 1969, 60B, 1—10
Burghardt, E., and *F. Bajardi:* Ergebnisse der Früherfassung des Kollumkarzinoms mittels Zytologie und Kolposkopie (Results obtained from Early Detection of Cervical Carcinoma by Cytological and Colposcopic Approaches). Arch. Gynäk. 1987 (1956), 621
Burghardt, E.: Über die atypische Umwandlungszone (Atypical Transformation Zone) Geburtsh. u. Frauenheilk. 19 (1959), 676—683
Burghardt, E., and *E. Holzer:* Die Lokalisation des pathologischen Zervixepithels (Localisation of Pathologically Affected Cervical Epithelium). Arch. Gynäk. 209 (1970), 305—330
Coppleson, M.: Die Stellung der Kolposkopie bei der Entdeckung und Behandlung des Ca in situ der Zervix (Role of Colposcopy in Detection and Treatment of Cervical Carcinoma in Situ). J. Obstet. Gynec. Brit. Comm. 71 (1964), 854
Coppleson, M.: Colposcopy, Cervical Carcinoma in Situ and the Gynaecologist, J. Obstet. Gynec. Brit. Comm. 71 (1964), 854
Coppleson, M., and *B. Reid:* Preclinical Carcinoma of the Cervix Uteri, Pergamon Press, Oxford, London, Edinburgh, New York, Toronto, Sydney, Paris, Braunschweig (1967)
Coppleson, M.: The Origin and Nature of Premalignant Lesions of the Cervix Uteri, Intern. J. Gynaec. Obstet. 8 (1970), 4, P.s.
Coppleson, M., *E. Pixley* and *B. Reid:* Colposcopy — A Scientific and Practical Approach to the Cervix in Health and Disease, Charles C. Thomas Publishers, Springfield I 11 (1971)
Coupez, F.: Sobse el luger que occupa la colposcopia en el examen ginecologico (Role played by Colposcopy in Gynaecological Examination). Progresos de Obstet. Ginecol. XI (1968), 331—342
Coupez, F.: La place de la colposcopie dans l'examen gynécologique actuel (Present Position of Colposcopy in Gynaecological Examination). Rev. franc. Gynéc. 56 (1970), 209—217
Cramer, H., and *G. Schulte:* Kolposkopische Fotografie im Agfa-Color-Negativ-Positiv-Verfahren (Use of Agfa-Color Negative-Positive Process for Colposcopic Photography). (1953), 212—216
Cramer, H.: Die Kolposkopie in der Praxis (Colposcopy in Practice) Georg Thieme Verlag, Stuttgart (1956).
Cramer, H.: Kritisches zum Begriff der sogenannten atypischen Umwandlungszone (Critical Appraisal of the Definition of Atypical Transformation Zone) Geburtsh. u. Frauenheilk. 21 (1961), 706—712
Davidson, C., and *Ch. W. Taylor:* A Study of Patients Previously Treated for In Situ Carcinoma of the Cervix, J. Obstet. Gynaecol. Brit. Comm. 80 (1973) 7, 654
Dietel, H., and *A. Focken:* Das Schicksal des atypischen Epithels an der Portio (Destiny of Atypical Portio Epithelium). Geburtsh. u. Frauenheilk. 15 (1955), 593—606
Dohnai, V.: Schwangerschaft und Schleimhautveränderungen an der Cervix uteri (Pregnancy and Alterations of Mucous Membrane in Cervix Uteri). Geburtsh. u. Gynäkol. Bd. 22/1 (1967), 4
Elsner, H.: Zur kolposkopisch atypischen Umwandlungszone (Atypical Transformation Zone in Colposcopy). Zbl. f. Gynäkol. A9 85/3 (1965), 1357 to 1361
Eschbach, W., and *W. Brucker:* Betrachtungen zur Genese und Klinik des Carcinoma colli uteri (Genesis and Clinical Pattern of Cervical Carcinoma). Dtsch. Gesundh.-Wesen 15 (1960), 1243—1247
Eschbach, W., *R. Huber* and *U. Bergmann:* Gegenwartsfragen der Diagnostik, Ausbreitung und Therapie des Zervixkarzinoms und seiner Vorstufen (Topical Issues relating to Diagnosis, Proliferation and Therapy of Cervical Carcinoma and Its Premalignant Stages). Arch. Geschwulstforsch. 41 (1973) 4, 336—358
Eschbach, W., and *U. Bergmann:* Gegenwartsfragen zum Carcinoma cervicis uteri (Topical Issues relating to Cervical Carcinoma). Dtsch. Gesundh.-Wes. No. 49, 29 (1974), 2305—2313
Eschbach, W., and *U. Bergmann:* Gegenwartsfragen zum Carcinoma cervicis uteri (Topical Issues relating to Cervical Carcinoma). Dtsch. Gesundh.-Wes. 29 (1974), 1361—1366
Eschbach, W.: Gegenwartsfragen zum Carcinoma cervicis uteri, 3. Mitteilung (Topical Issues relating to Cervical Carcinoma, Third communication). Dtsch. Gesundh.-Wes. 31 (1976), 17
Fanghänel, M.: Kolposkopie und Zytologie — unentbehrliches Hilfsmittel bei der Krebsfährtensuche auch kleinerer gynäkologischer Kliniken (Colposcopy and Cytology — Tools Indispensable even to Smaller Gynaecological Units in Tracking Down Cancer). Zschr. ärztl. Fortbild. 62, 12, 666
Fernandes, M.: Epithelveränderungen am Collum uteri während der Gravidität (Changes to Cervical Epithelium during Gravidity). Rev. Chincc. Obstet. (Rio de Janeiro) 108 (1961), 227—264
Fischel, W.: Beiträge zur Morphologie der Portio

vaginalis uteri (Morphology of Portio Veginalis Uteri). Arch. Gynäkol. 16 (1880), 192

Fluhmann, C. F.: The Histogenesis of Acquired Erosions of the Cervix Uteri, Am. J. Obstet. Gynecol. 82 (1961), 970

Frankel, P. E.: Leukoplakie, Leukoplakie — Grund und Gedanken zur Pathogenese (Leucoplakia, Leucoplakia — Floor — Reflections on Pathogenesis). Dtsch. med. J. 11 (1960) 6, 134—136

Frankel, P. E.: Die Kolposkopie im Dienste der Gynäkologie (Colposcopy in the Service of Gynaecology) Dtsch. med. J. 11 (1960) 11, 358—360.

Friedmann, H. P.: The Use of Ultraviolet Light and Fluorescent Dyes in the Detection of Uterine Cancer by Vaginal Smear, Am. J. Obstet. Gynecol. 59 (1950), 852

Fritsch, K.: Über Endozervixkolposkopie (Endocervical Colposcopy), ref. (reviewed) in Geburtsh. u. Frauenheilk. 19 (1959), 64

Ganse, R.: Atypische Gefäßentwicklung beim Portiokarzinom (Atypical Vascularisation in Concomitance with Portio Carcinoma). Zbl. Gynäkol. 19 (1952), 749

Ganse, R.: Die Bedeutung der Relationspathologie für die kolposkopische Weiterentwicklung (Relativity Pathology — Its Bearings on Progress in Colposcopy). Z. Geburtsh. Gynäkol. 1 (1952), 137

Ganse, R.: Kolpophotogramme zur Einführung in die Kolposkopie (Colpophotograms for Introduction to Colposcopy). Akademie-Verlag, Berlin (1953)

Ganse, R.: Vertiefung der Kolposkopie (Improvement of Colposcopy). Zbl. Gynäkol. 34a (1954), 1541—1551

Ganse, R.: Über das schnelle Entstehen von gesteigert atypischem Epithel auf dem Boden einer Ektopie (Rapid Formation of Increasingly Atypical Epithelium on the Basis of Ectopy). Oncologia 28, III (1955) 4, 232—233

Ganse, R.: Über die Bedeutung der Gefäßveränderung beim Portiokarzinom (Role of Vascular Change in Portio Carcinoma). An. bras. ginecol. 40 (1955), 155—163

Ganse, R.: Zur Pathogenese des Portiokarzinoms und Erleichterung seiner Frühdiagnose durch farbige Kolpofotogramme, III. Bd. mit farbigen Kolpofotogrammen in Kassette (Pathogenesis of Portio Carcinoma and Facilitated Early Diagnosis by Use of Coloured Colpophotograms, III. Vol. with box of coloured colpophotograms). Akademie-Verlag, Berlin 1955

Ganse, R.: Beobachtung über rasche Rückbildung eines atypischen Epithels an der Portio (Observation of Soon Regression of Atypical Portio Epithelium). Zbl. Gynäkol. 8, 78/1 (1956), 314—317

Ganse, R.: Die Erleichterung der Frühdiagnose des Portiokarzinoms durch die erweiterte Kolposkopie (Early Diagnosis of Portio Carcinoma facilitated by Extended Colposcopy). Zschr. ärztl. Fortbild. 52 (1958) 2, 64—67

Ganse, R.: Das normale und pathologische Gefäßbild der Portio vaginalis uteri (Normal and Pathological Vascular Pattern of Portio Vaginalis Uteri). Akademie-Verlag, Berlin (1958)

Ganse, R.: Gefäßneubildung beim präinvasiven und fertigen Karzinom (Neovascularisation in Pre-Invasive and Manifest Carcinoma) Geburtsh. u. Frauenheilk. 20 (1960), 694—697

Ganse, R.: Kolposkopische und zytologische Studien in zwangloser Folge (Random Selection of Colposcopic and Cytological Studies) Georg Thieme, Leipzig, No. 7 (1961)

Ganse, R., R. Krimmenau and *J. Brey:* Papillomatöse Veränderungen der Portio und deren karzinomatöse Potenz (Papillomatous Alterations of the Portio — Their Carcinomatous Potential). Geburtsh. u. Frauenheilk. 22 (1962), 232—243

Ganse, R.: Einführung in die Kolposkopie (Introduction to Colposcopy-. Gustav-Fischer-Verlag, Jena (1963)

Ganse, R.: Veränderungen der atypischen Gefäße des Portiokarzinoms unter Telekobaltbestrahlung (Change in Atypical Vessels of Portio Carcinoma in Response to Tele-Cobalt Irradiation). Geburtsh. u. Frauenheilk. 27 (1967), 476—480

Gedigk, P., R. Müller and *H. Bechtelsheimer:* Nomenklatur und Einteilung gutartiger, präkanzeröser und maligner Veränderungen an der Cervix uteri (Nomenclature and Subdivision of Benign, Precancerous, and Malignant Changes in the Cervix Uteri). Beitr. Pathol. 147 (1972) 1, 57

Gerli, M., and *D. Berlingieri:* Die kombinierte Anwendung der Kolpozytologie und der Kolposkopie in der Frühdiagnose des Kollumkarzinoms (Combined Use of Colpocytology and Colposcopy in Early Diagnosis of Cervical Carcinoma). Minerva ginec. (Torino) 14 (1962), 539—552

Gillet, J. Y., G. Rihm, J. G. Koritke et al.: Vascularisation of the Cervix Uteri in Women, Rev. Fr. Gynecol. Obstet. 68 (1973) 1, 13—24

Glatthaar, E.: Leukoplakie und Plattenepithelkarzinom der Portio (Leukoplakia and Squamous Cell Carcinoma of the Portio). Wschr. Geburtsh. 120 (1945), 33

Glatthaar, E.: Die Regenerationsvorgänge an der Portio und ihre Bedeutung für die Entstehung des Kollumkarzinoms (Processes of Regeneration in the Portio — Bearings on Pathogenesis of Cervical Carcinoma). Gynaecologia 128 (1949), 29

Glatthaar, E.: Die Vor- und Frühstadien des Portiokarzinoms (Premalignant and Early Phases of Portio Carcinoma). Oncologia V (1952), 196

Glatthaar, E.: Kolposkopie (Biologie und Pathologie des Weibes — Ein Handbuch der Frauenheilkunde und der Geburtshilfe) (Colposcopy — Biology and Pathology of Women — Handbook of Gynaecology and Obstetrics). Vol. III, 1955, Verlag Urban & Schwarzenberg

Gonzalez-Merlo, J., J. Ausin, J. A. Lejarcegui et al.: Regeneration of the Ectocervical Epithelium after Its Destruction by Electrocauterisation, Acta Cytol. 17 (1973), 4, 366

Gray, I. A.: Dysplasia, Carcinoma in Situ, and Micro-Invasive Carcinoma of the Cervix, Springfield, Thomas 1964

Greggersen, C., and *K. Semm:* Kolposkopische und histologische Verlaufskontrollen der thermo-koag lierten gutartigen Portioveränderungen (Colposcopic and Histological Follow-Up Checks of Thermo-Coagulated Benign Portio Changes). Geb. Fra. **32** (1972), 671–677

Gruenagel, H. H.: Die Plattenepithel-Zylinderepithel-Grenze an der Portio vaginalis uteri bei unreifen und reifen neugeborenen Säuglingen und Kindern bis zu neun Jahren (Boundary between Squamous and Columnar Epithelia of Portio Vaginalis Uteri in Immature and Mature Newborn and in Children up to Nine Years Old). Frankfurt. Z. Path. **68** (1957), 465

Guhr, O.: Kolposkopische, zytologische und histologische Portiobefunde bei ovulationshemmenden Medikamenten (Colposcopic, Cytological, and Histological Portio Findings obtained from Women on Ovulation Inhibitors). Arch. Gynäkol. **202** (1965), 205–207

Guhr, O.: Portioveränderungen unter Kortikosteroiden (Portio Changes in Response to Corticosteroids). Münch. med. Wschr. **115** (1973), 1020–1022

Hamperl, H., C. Kaufmann, K. G. Ober and *P. Schneppenheim:* Die „Erosion" der Portio — Die Entstehung der Pseudoerosion, das Ektropion und die Plattenepithelüberhäutung der Zervixdrüsen auf der Portiooberfläche ("Erosion" of the Portio — Genesis of Pseudo-Erosion, Ectropion, and Squamous Epithelium Epidermisation of Cervical Glands on Portio Surface). Virchows Archiv **331** (1958), 51–71

Hamperl, H.: Die angeborene Pseudoerosion der Portio und ihr Schicksal (Innate Pseudo-Erosion of Portio — Prognosis). Arch. Gynäkol. **200** (1965), 299

Held, E.: Intrazervikale Lokalisation des nichtinvasiven, atypischen Pflasterepithels und des beginnenden Pflasterzellkarzinoms (Intracervical Localisation of Non-Invasive, Atypical Squamous Epithelium and Incipient Squamous Cell Carcinoma). Arch. Gynäkol. 188 (1957) 3, 376–390

Hillemanns, H. G.: Entstehung und Wachstum des Zervixkarzinoms (Genesis and Growth of Cervical Carcinoma). S. Karger — Basle, New York, 1964

Hillemanns, H. G., J. E. Ayre and *J. M. Le Guerrier:* Die Einwirkung von Steroiden auf Krebsvorstadien an der Zervix (Action of Steroids on Premalignant Stages in the Cervix). Arzneimittelforschg. **14** (1964), 784–791

Hinselmann, H.: Handbuchkapitel in Veit-Stoeckel 6/I, S. 888 — Diagnose des Portiokarzinoms nebst Frühdiagnose (Chapter in Veit-Stoeckel Handbook 6/I, p. 888 — Diagnosis of Portio Carcinoma, including Early Diagnosis)

Hinselmann, H.: Verbesserung der Inspektionsmöglichkeiten von Vulva, Vagina und Portio (Improvement of Possibilities for Inspection of Vulva, Vagina, and Portio). Münch. med. Wschr. **72** (1925), 1733

Hinselmann, H.: Zur Kenntnis der präkanzerösen Veränderung der Portio (Knowledge on Precancerous Change of Portio). Zbl. Gynäkol. **51 I** (1927) 901–903

Hinselmann, H.: Der Begriff der Umwandlungszone der Portio (Notion of Transformation Zone of Portio). Arch. Gynäkol. **131** (1927), 422–424

Hinselmann, H.: Das klinische Bild der indirekten Metaplasie der ektopischen Zylinderzellenschleimhaut der Portio (Clinical Pattern of Indirect Metaplasia of Ectopic Columnar Cell Mucous Membrane of the Portio). Arch. Gynäkol. **133** (1928), 64–69

Hinselmann, H.: Die klinische Frühdiagnose des Portio-Ca (Clinical Early Diagnosis of Portio Carcinoma). Zbl. Gynäkol. 52 III (1928), 2797–2798

Hinselmann, H.: Felderung der Scheidenhaut (Field Pattern of Vaginal Mucous Membrane). Zschr. Geburtsh. u. Gynäkol. **101** (1932), 166–183

Hinselmann, H.: Die klinische Differenzierung der Matrixbezirke (Clinical Differentiation of Matrix Regions). Zbl. Gynäkol. (1933) 29, 1682

Hinselmann, H.: Ausgewählte Gesichtspunkte zur Beurteilung des Zusammenhanges der „Matrixbezirke" des Ca der sichtbaren Abschnitte des weiblichen Genitaltraktes (Selected Aspects for Assessment of Relationship between "Matrix Regions" of Carcinoma of Visible Parts of Female Genital Tract). Zschr. Geburtsh. **104** (1933), 228–243

Hinselmann, H.: Der Begriff der Prämatrix (Notion of Prematrix). Zbl. Gynäkol. **41** (1933), 2402–2406

Hinselmann, H.: Die klinische mikroskopische Frühdiagnose (Clinical Microscopic Early Diagnosis). Arch. Gynäkol. **156** (1933), 239–244

Hinselmann, H.: Einführung in die Kolposkopie (Introduction to Colposcopy). Paul Hartung Verlag, Hamburg (1933)

Hinselmann, H.: Die Essigsäureprobe, ein Bestandteil der erweiterten Kolposkopie (Acetic Acid Test, Part of Extended Colposcopy). Dtsch. med. Wschr. **40** (1938)

Hinselmann, H.: Die Leistungsfähigkeit der modernen Frühdiagnose des Ca am Muttermund (Potentiality, Today, of Early Diagnosis of Carcinoma of Os Uteri). Dtsch. med. Wschr. **65** (1939), 954–957

Hinselmann, H.: Der Nachweis der aktiven Ausgestaltung der Gefäße beim jungen Portiokarzinom als neues differential-diagnostisches Hilfsmittel (Determination of Vascular Activity at Early Stages of Portio Carcinoma — A New Tool in Differential Diagnosis). Zbl. Gynäkol. **64** (1940), 1810

Hinselmann, H.: Über die Geschichte der Kolposkopie (History of Colposcopy). Z. ärztl. Fortb. **46** (1952), 702–731

Hinselmann, H., and *A. Schütt:* Die Kolposkopie (Colposcopy). Verlag W. Girardet, Wuppertal-Elberfeld 1954

Hinselmann, H.: Die Kolposkopie, mit einem Beitrag über die Kolpofotografie (Colposcopy, including a contribution on Colpophotography). W. Girardet, Wuppertal 1954

Hinselmann, H.: Gibt es Vorstadien des Portio-Ca? (Are there Premalignant Stages of Portio Carcinoma?) Medizinische **1** (1955), 116–117

Hinselmann, H.: Janusgrün, ein wertvolles Färbemittel in der modernen Kolposkopie (Janus Green, A Useful Dye in Modern Colposcopy). Laboratoriumsblätter Behringwerke 22–24, 1958

Hinselmann, H.: Kolposkopische Studien in zwangloser Folge (Random Selection of Colposcopic Studies). Verlag Georg Thieme, Leipzig, No. 1 — 1954, No. 2 — 1956, No. 3 — 1957, No. 4 — 1958, No. 5 — 1959, No. 6 — 1960

Hirschberg, H. K.: Erleichterung der Kolposkopie (How to Facilitate Colposcopic Examination). Zbl. Gynäkol. (1939), 2306

Hohlbein, R.: Lokalisation der kolposkopischen Hauptbefunde bei gesteigert atypischem Epithel und Mikrokarzinom (Lokalisation of Major Colposcopic Findings relating to Increasingly Atypical Epithelium and Microcarcinoma). Zbl. Gynäkol. **80**/2 (1958) 19, 738—743

Hohlbein, R., and *R. Krimmenau*: Die intrazervikale Lokalisation des gesteigert atypischen Epithels und des Mikrokarzinoms (Intracervical Localisation of Increasingly Atypical Epithelium and Microcarcinoma). Geburtsh. u. Frauenheilk. **8**, 18/2 (1958), 1030—1042

Hohlbein, R.: Die Fluoreszenz-Kolposkopie und Fluoreszenz-Kolpofotografie (Fluorescent Colposcopy and Fluorescent Colpophotography). Geburtsh. u. Frauenheilk. **19** (1959), 656—669

Holtorff, J.: Über die Leistungsfähigkeit der Kolposkopie bei der Früherkennung des Kollumkarzinoms (Performance Potential of Colposcopy in Early Detection of Cervical Carcinoma). Ztschr. ärztl. Fortb. **51** (1957) 16, 670—676

Holtorff, J.: Über das Schicksal des einfach atypischen Epithels (Hinselmann) an der Portio (Prognosis of Simple Atypical Epithelium (Hinselmann) of the Portio). Zbl. Gynäkol. (1958) 37

Holtorff, J.: Kolposkopische Kriterien der atypischen Umwandlungszone (Colposcopic Criteria of Atypical Transformation Zone). Geburtsh. u. Frauenheilk. **20** (1960), 931—941

Holtorff, J.: Beitrag zur kolposkopischen Gefäßdiagnostik an der Portio (Colposcopic Examination of Portio Vessels). Gynaecologia **151** (1961), 417—427

Hollyock, V. E., and *W. Chanen*: The use of the colposcope in the selection of patients for cervical cone biopsy, Am. J. Obstet. Gynecol. **114** (1972) 2, 185

Janisch, H., and *Chr. Lanik*: Über den didaktischen Wert der kolposkopischen Gruppeneinteilung (Didactic Usefulness of Colposcopic Grouping). Münch. med. Wschr. **20** (1962), 933—935

Johannisson, E., *P. Kolstad* and *G. Soederberg*: Cytologic, Vascular, and Histologic Patterns of Dysplasia, Carcinoma in Situ, and Early Invasive Carcinoma of the Cervix, Acta Radiologico Supplementum 258, Stockholm 1966

Kaiser, P.: Kolposkopische, zytologische und histologische Portiobefunde bei Antikonzeptionsbehandlung mit Ovosiston (Colposcopic, Cytological, and Histological Portio Findings recorded from Women on Ovosiston Contraceptive). Zbl. Gynäkol. **92** (1970), 401—404

Käser, O., *V. Friedberg*, *K. G. Ober*, *K. Thomsen* and *J. Zander*: Gynäkologie und Geburtshilfe, Band III — Spezielle Gynäkologie (Gynaecology and Obstetrics, Volume III — Specialised Gynaecology). Georg-Thieme-Verlag Stuttgart (1972)

Kalbfleisch, H. H.: Die Relationspathologie Gustav Rickers als Grundlage der Krankheitslehre (Gustav Ricker's Relativity Pathology — A Foundation of Nosology). Dtsch. med. Wschr. (1948) 47/48, 625—628

Kaufmann, C.: Früherkennung des Kollumkarzinoms (Early Detection of Cervical Carcinoma). Springer-Verlag, Berlin, Göttingen, Heidelberg 1957

Kaufmann, C.: Epithelveränderungen der Zervix (Alterations in Cervical Epithelium). Zbl. Gynäkol. 14 (1957), 555

Kern, G., and *J. Zander*: Gefäßveränderungen im Verlauf der Karzinogenese (Vascular Change in the Course of Carcinogenesis). Z. Krebsforsch. **63** (1959), 168—183

Kern, G., and *H. P. Bötzelen*: Kolposkopischer Befund und Lokalisation des Carcinoma in situ (Colposcopic Findings and Localisation of Carcinoma in Situ). Arch. Gynäkol. **194** (1961), 564—585

Kern, G.: Carcinoma in Situ, Springer-Verlag, Heidelberg, New York, Berlin 1964

Kern, G., *E. Rissmann* and *G. Hund*: Die Leistungsfähigkeit der Kolposkopie bei der Frühdiagnostik des Kollumkarzinoms (Performance Potential of Colposcopy in Early Diagnosis of Cervical Carcinoma). Arch. Gynäkol. **199** (1964), 526

Kirsch, R., and *G. Rieck*: Das Verhalten der Blutgefäße beim Karzinom der Mamma und der Portio uteri (Behaviour of Blood Vessels in Conjunction with Mammary and Uterine Portio Carcinomas). Zschr. ärztl. Fortb. **11** (1954), 384, 388/389

Koč, J., *V. Mikolas* and *V. Lané*: Das Bild des terminalen Blutgefäßnetzes auf der karzinomatösen Cervix uteri (Pattern of Terminal Blood Vessel Network on Carcinomatous Uterine Cervix). Zbl. Gynäkol. (1960), 39

Koller, O.: Kolpofotografischu undersokelsev ar karvorholdene ved cancer cervicis uteri (Colpophotographic Examination of Cervical Carcinoma). Forh. Nord. Foren. Obstet. Gynek. Kongr. Oslo 1956, 123—126

Koller, O.: The Vascular Patterns of the Uterine Cervix, Scand. Univ. Books Universitetsforlaget A. W. Broggers Boktr. Oslo (1963)

Koller, O., and *T. Kolstad*: Die Bedeutung des kolposkopischen Gefäßbildes beim Zervixkarzinom (Relevance of Colposcopically Recorded Vascular Pattern to Assessment of Cervical Carcinoma). GBK Mitteilungsdienst 5 (1969), 495—511

Kolstad, P.: Vascularisation, Oxygen Tension, and Radiocurability in Cancer of the Cervix, Universitetsforlaget, Copenhagen (1963)

Kolstad, P.: The Colposcopic Picture of Trichomonas Vaginitis, Acta Obstet. Gynec. Scand. **43** (1964), 388

Kolstad, P.: Colposcopic Diagnosis of Dysplasia, Carcinoma in Situ, and Early Invasive Cancer of the Cervix, Acta Obstet. Gynec. Scand. **43**, Suppl. 7 (1964), 105—108

Kolstad, P.: Carcinoma of the Cervix, Stage 0, Am. J. Obstet. Gynec. **96** (1966), 1098–1111

Kolstad, P., and *A. Stafl*: Atlas of Colposcopy, Universitetsforlaget, Oslo (1972)

Kopecny, J.: Die Gefäßzeichnung der Cervix uteri im kolpomikroskopischen Bild (Colpomicroscopic Representation of Cervical Vessels). Zbl. Gynäkol. **36** (1967), 1324–1328

Kos, J.: Gefäßanordnung in der Portio vaginalis cervicis uteri unter normalem gesunden Plattenepithel (Arrangement of Vessels in Portio Vaginalis Cervicis Uteri beneath Normal, Clinically Intact Squamous Epithelium). Zbl. Gynäkol. **82** (1960), 1849–1855

Kos, J.: Darstellung der Gefäßkapillaren an Exzisionen aus der Cervix uteri auf histochemischem Wege (Histochemical Representation of Vascular Capillaries in Material Excised from the Uterine Cervix). Zbl. Gynäkol. **84** (1962), 538–541

Kos, J., and *V. Lane*: Die Gefäße des Terminalblutnetzes und der Portio vaginalis (Vessels of Terminal Network at Vaginal Portio). Cs. Cynekol. **27/41** (1962), 220–223

Kraatz, H.: Farbfiltervorschaltung zur leichteren Erlernung der Kolposkopie (Use of Colour Filters for More Convenient Training in Colposcopy). Zbl. Gynäkol. **63** (1939), 2307–2309

Kratochwil, A., and *G. Tatra*: Über den Malignitätsindex kolposkopischer Atypien (Malignancy Index of Colposcopic Atypias). Wien. med. Wschr. (1060) 46, 785–787

Kreyberg, L.: Über präkanzeröse Gefäßveränderungen (Precancerous Vascular Changes). Virchows Arch. path. Anat. Physiologie, Berlin, Springer-Verlag **273** (1929)

Krüger, E. H.: Über die Kolposkopie und die Möglichkeiten ihrer Erlernung (Colposcopy and Possible Ways to Learn Its Use). Med. Klin. **52** (1957), 1781–1788

Krüger, E. H.: Über das Gefäßbild beim beginnenden Karzinom (Vascular Pattern of Incipient Carcinoma). Zbl. Gynäkol. **43** (1957), 1669

Krüger, E. H.: Über die Topographie koposkopischer Befunde und histologischer Epithelveränderungen an der Portio uteri (Topography of Colposcopically and Histologically Recorded Changes in Epithelium of the Uterine Portio). Zbl. Gynäkol. **79**, 2 (1957) 20, 789–796

Krüger, E. H.: Praktische Kolposkopie, Teil I (Colposcopic Practice, Part I) Med. Klin. **55** (1960) 45, 2006–2008

Kyriazis, G. A., *H. Balin* and *R. L. Lipson*: Haematoporphyrin-Derivative-Fluorescence Test Colposcopy and Colpophotography in the Diagnosis of Atypical Metaplasia, Dysplasia, and Carcinoma in Situ of the Cervix Uteri, Am. J. Obstet. Gynecol. **117** (1973) 3, 375

Lane, V.: Der Verlauf der Epithelisierung der Portio vaginalis nach der Elektrothermokoagulation und ihre Bedeutung für die Vorbeugung des Karzinoms (Course of Epithelisation of the Vaginal Portio, following Electrothermocoagulation — Its Importance to Carcinoma Prophylaxis). Gynaecology, **149** (1960) 2, 89–97

Lang, W. R., and *A. E. Rakoff*: Colposcopy and Cytology, Obstetrics and Gynaecology **8** (1956) 3, 312–317

Lang, W. R.: Colposcopy-Neglected Method of Cervical Evaluation, J. Am. med. Ass. **166/2** (1958) 8, 893–897

Lax, H.: Das Oberflächenkarzinom (Surface Carcinoma). Z. Geb. u. Gynäkol. **138** (1953), 105

Leeb, H., and *R. Ulm*: Das präklinische Carcinoma colli uteri (Preclinical Cervical Carcinoma). Gynaecologia, **149** (1960) 2, 81–89

Leip, F.: Krebsbekämpfung und Kolposkopie (Control of Cancer and Colposcopy). Med. Welt 8 (1936)

Limburg, H.: Die Frühdiagnose des Uteruskarzinoms (Early Diagnosis of Uterus Carcinoma). 3rd ed., G. Thieme, Stuttgart (1956)

Linhartova, A., and *A. Stafl*: Zur Morphologie des Ektropiums an der Portio vaginalis uteri (Morphololy of Ectropion at Portio Vaginalis Uteri). Arch. Gynäkol. **200** (1964), 131–141

Lundström, P., and *E. Segerbrand*: Therapeutische Resultate der kolposkopisch kontrollierten Entnahme von Kollumgewebe bei atypischem Zellabstrich der Frauen im Alter bis zu 35 Jahren (Sampling of Cervical Tissue from Women up to 35 Years with Atypical Cell Smear under Colposcopic Control — Therapeutic Results). Zbl. Gynäkol. **97** (1975) 8, 449–455

Madej, J.: Die Anwendung der Milchsäurelösung als Kontrastmittel in der erweiterten Kolposkopie (Use of Lactic Acid Solution as a Contrast Medium in Extended Colposcopy). Geburtsh. u. Frauenheilk. **22** (1962), 1427–1432

Madej, J.: Angio-Architecture of Sub-Epithelial Blood Vessels in Colposcopically Unsuspicious Portio Erythroplakia, Gynaecologia, Basle **164** (1967), 283

Madej, J.: Place of Colposcopy in Early Detection of Uterine Cervix Neoplasma, Ginekologia Polska **43** (1972) 11, 1277

Majewski, A.: Die Nor-Adrenalinprobe als neues Hilfsmittel der Kolposkopie (Noradrenaline Test — A New Approach in Support of Colposcopy). Geburtsh. u. Frauenheilk. **20** (1960), 983–988

Majewski, A., and *A. Platen*: Kolposkopische Befunde beim Carcinoma in situ und Mikrokarzinom am Collum uteri — Erwiderung auf die Arbeit „Kolposkopische Befunde und Lokalisation des Carcinoma in situ" von G. *Kern* und H. P. *Bötzelen* (Colposcopic Findings Recordable from Carcinoma in Situ and Microcarcinoma of the Uterine Cervix — Reply to a Paper published by G. *Kern* and H. P. *Bötzelen* under the Heading of "Colposcopic Findings and Localisation of Carcinoma in Situ"). Arch. Gynäkol. **196** (1962), 629–633

Margitay-Becht, D.: Kolposkopische Untersuchungen bei schwangeren und sterilen Frauen (Colposcopic Examination of Pregnant and Sterile Women). Zbl. Gynäkol. **82** (1960), 1193–1198

Menken, F.: Fotokolposkopie und Foto-Douglaskopie (Photocolposcopy and Photo-Douglascopy). W. Giradet, Wuppertal-Elberfeld 1955

Mestwerdt, G.: Zur histologischen Beurteilung kolposkopischer Bilder (Histological Assessment of Colposcopic Findings). Arch. Gynäkol. **166** (1938), 316

Mestwerdt, G.: Atlas der Kolposkopie (Atlas of Colposcopy). Fischer, Jena 1949/1953

Mestwerdt, G., and *H. J. Wespi*: Atlas der Kolposkopie (Atlas of Colposcopy), 3rd ed., Fischer, Stuttgart 1961

Mestwerdt, G., and *H. J. Wespi*: Atlas der Kolposkopie (Atlas of Colposcopy), 6th ed., Fischer-Verlag, Stuttgart 1974

Meyer, R.: Die Epithelentwicklung der Cervix und Portio vaginalis uteri und die Pseudoerosio congenita (Development of Epithelium in Cervix and Portio and Congenital Pseudo-Erosion). Arch. Gynäkol. **91** (1910), 579

Mikolas, V., *A. Stafl* and *A. Linhartova*: Das terminale Gefäßbild der Portio vaginalis uteri bei Schwangeren (Terminal Vessels of the Portio Vaginalis Uteri in the Pregnant Woman). Zbl. Gynäkol. **84** (1962), 524–538

Mikolas, V., *H. Stafl* and *A. Linhartova*: The Terminal Vascular Network of the Uterine Cervix in Physiological Conditions and in Precancer, Acta Un. Int. Cancer **20** (1964), 729

Mikolas, V., *A. Stafl*, *J. Mleziva* and *A. Linhartova*: Veränderungen des terminalen Gefäßnetzes der Scheide bei Kolpitis (Changes in the Terminal Vascular Rete of the Vagina in the Pressence of Colpitis). Zbl. Gynäkol. **86** (1964), 701

v. Mikulicz-Radecki, F.: Können Vorsichtsuntersuchungen und Krebsberatungsstellen die Früherfassung der Genitalkarzinome fördern? (Can Early Detection of Genital Carcinomas be facilitated by Prophylactic Examinations and Cancer Briefing Centres?) Arch. Gynäkol. **189** (1957), 336–343

Muth, H.: Vergleichende zytologisch-Kolposkopische Untersuchungen (Comparative Cytologico-Colposcopic Examinations). Geburtsh. u. Frauenheilk. 10, **15.2** (1955), 907–916

Muth, H.: Zur Frühdiagnostik des Kollumkarzinoms (Early Diagnosis of Cervical Carcinoma). Zbl. Gynäkol. 46, 78/4 (1956), 1825–1829

Muth, H.: Die Bedeutung der Kolposkopie und Zytologie für die Frühdiagnostik des Kollumkarzinoms (Relevance of Colposcopy and Cytology to Early Diagnosis of Cervical Carcinoma). Dtsch. Med. Welt **43** (1965), 2414–2417

Nold, B.: Über die atypische Umwandlungszone der Portio — Das kolposkopische Bild (Atypical Transformation Zone of the Portio — Colposcopic Representation). Med. Bild **3** (1960)

Navratil, E.: Colposcopy, Charles C. Thomas, Springfield, Ill., USA 1964

Naujoks, H.: Diagnostische Probleme der Früherkennung. I. Teil — Gynäkologie (Diagnostic Problems of Early Detection. Part I — Gynaecology). **1** (1969) 4, 166–173

Nunes-Montiel, J. T.: Colposcopy as a Method of Exploring the Endocervix, Rev. Obstet. ginec. Venes. **26** (1966), 431

Ober, K. G., *P. Schneppenheim*, *H. Hamperl* and *C. Kaufmann*: Die Epithelgrenzen im Bereich des Isthmus uteri (Epithelial Boundaries in the Uterine Isthmus Region). Arch. Gynäkol. **190** (1958), 346–383

Ober, K. G.: Cervix uteri und Lebensalter (Uterine Cervix and Age). Dtsch. med. Wschr. **83** (1958), 1661

Olson, A. W., and *E. E. Nichols*: Leucoplakia of the Cervix — Mosaic and Papillary Pattern, Am. J. Obstet. & Gynecol. 82 (1961) 4, 895–902

Oudkerk, P. M.: De diagnose van het carcinoma colli uteri (Diagnosis of Cervical Carcinoma). Ned. T. v. Verlosk. en Gyn. 57 (1957), 411

Padovec, J., *J. Kanka* and *J. Subrt*: Prevention of Cancer of the Uterine Cervix, Intern. Surg. **51** (1969), 443–449

Pfleiderer, A.: Kapillarmikroskopische Beobachtungen der Portio und Vagina (Microscopic Inspection of Portio and Vaginal Capillaries). Verl. Dtsch. Ges. Gynäkol. 22 (1931), 595

Preissecker, E.: Das kolposkopische Bild der karzinomatösen Beläge (Colposcopic Representation of Carcinomatous Coats). Wien. klin. Wschr. (1929) 1352

Rassler, R.: Der Ausstoßungsmechanismus des Menstruationsblutes unter dem Kolposkop — Inaugural Diss. (Colposcopic Representation of the Mechanism of Menstruation Blood Ejection — Inaugural Dissertation). Jena (1950)

Ribbert, H.: Über das Gefäßsystem und die Heilbarkeit der Geschwülste (Vascular System and Curability of Tumours). Dtsch. med. Wschr. **30** (1904), 801–803

Ricker, G.: Relationspathologie — Pathologie als Naturwissenschaft (Relativity Pathology — Pathology as a Science). Springer-Verlag 1924

Rieck, G.: Über die praktische und wissenschaftliche Bedeutung der Vorsorgeuntersuchung zur Früherfassung und Prophylaxe des Portiokarzinoms (Theoretical and Pratical Importance of Prophylactic Examination to Early Detection and Prophylaxis of Portio Carcinoma). Z. ärztl. Fortb. **1** (1954) 17

Rocha, A. H.: Die Differentialdiagnostik kolposkopischer Befunde mit der Albothylprobe — Prophylaxe (Use of Albothyl Test for Differential Diagnosis of Colposcopic Findings). Zbl. Sozialhyg. Gesundheitsvor. Grenzgebiete **103** (1971), 37–43

Rummel, A.: Kolposkopische und zytologische Befunde während und nach Behandlung mit Gestagenen (Colposcopic and Cytological Findings during and after Gestagen Treatment). Geburtsh. u. Frauenheilk. **26** (1966), 593–596

Salzer, R. B.: Colposcopy — An Aid in the Detection of Early Cancer and Precancerous Conditions of the Cervix, Obstet. and Gynecol. **13** (1959), 4

Scheffey, L. C., *W. R. Lang* and *G. Tatarion*: An Experimental Program with Colposcopy, Am. J. Obstet. **70** (1955) 2, 876–888

von Scheidt, R. G.: Kolposkopie-Kursus (Course in Colposcopy). Blaschker Verlag, Berlin

Schiller, W.: Untersuchungen zur Entstehung der Geschwülste (Studies into the Genesis of Tumours). Virchows Archiv **263** (1927), 279

Schiller, W.: Zur klinischen Frühdiagnose des Portiokarzinoms (Early Clinical Diagnosis of Portio Carcinoma). Zbl. Gynäkol. **52** (1928), 1886

Schiller, W.: Jodpinselung und Abschabung des Portioepithels (Iodine Painting and Scraping of Portio Epithelium). Zbl. Gynäkol. (1929) 53, 1056

Schmitt, A.: Colposcopy, American Academy of General Practice, 98 (1964), 98–197

Schneppenheim, P., H. Hamperl, C. Kaufmann and *K. G. Ober:* Die Beziehungen des Schleimhautepithels zum Plattenepithel an der Cervix uteri im Lebenslauf der Frau (Relationships between Mucosal Epithelium and Squamous Epithelium in the Uterine Cervix during one Life Span). Arch Gynäkol. **190** (1958), 303

Scott, J. W., P. Brass and *D. Seckinger:* Colposcopy plus Cytology, Am. J. Obstet. Gynecol. **103** (1962), 336

Sebek, V., and *K. Vesely:* Ein Beitrag zur Kolposkopie während der Schwangerschaft — Kolposkopische und zytologische Studien in zwangloser Folge (Colposcopy during Pregnancy — Random Selection of Colposcopic and Cytological Studies). No. 8, Georg Thieme — Leipzig (1962)

Smakhtina, O. L., A. M. Aisurova, E. V. Isakova, et al.: Colposcopic and Cytological Studies in Pretumour and Malignant Changes in the Cervix Uteri, Voprosy onkologii (Russian) **21** (1975) 10, 45

Stafl, A., V. Dohnal and *A. Linhartova:* Kolposkopische, histologische und Gefäßbefunde an der krankhaft veränderten Portio (Colposcopic, Histological, and Vascular Findings obtained from Women with Pathologically Altered Portio). Geb. Fra. **23** (1963), 437–445

Stafl, A., A. Linhartova and *V. Dohnal:* Das kolposkopische Bild des papillären Grundes, der atypischen Umwandlungszone und deren Pathogenese (Colposcopic Representation of Papillary Floor, Atypical Transformation Zone, and their Pathogenesis). Arch. Gynäkol. **204** (1967) 212, reviewed in Geburtsh. u. Frauenheilk. **28** (1968), 893

Stafl, A., and *R. F. Mattingly:* Colposcopic Diagnosis of Cervical Neoplasia, Obstet. gynecol. **41** (1973), 168–176

Stafl, A., and *R. F. Mattingly:* Angiogenesis of Cervical Neoplasia, Am. J. Obstet. Gynecol. **121** (1975) 6, 845

Steffen, F. W.: Über die Leistungsfähigkeit der Kolposkopie in der gynäkologischen Sprechstunde (Relevance of Colposcopy to Gynaecological Consultation). Dtsch. Gesundh. Wes. No. 24/4 (1969) 41, 1961–1964

Stoeckel, W.: Die Kolposkopie, die Diagnose und die Therapie des Portiokarzinoms (Colposcopy, Diagnosis, and Therapy of Portio Carcinoma). Zbl. Gynäkol. (1942), 1590

Stoll, P., H. G. Bach and *M. Oppitz:* Die Portioerosion und ihre Bedeutung für die Frühdiagnostik des Karzinoms (Erosion of the Portio — Bearings on Early Diagnosis of Carcinoma). Dtsch. med. Wschr. **83** (1958) 4, 146–149

Sugihara, S.: The Morphological Study of Blood Vessels in Cervical Carcinoma, Acta Med. Okayma **12** (1958), 261–280

Tatra, G., and *A. Kratochwil:* Über den Malignitätsindex kolposkopischer Atypien (Malignancy Index of Colposcopic Atypias). Wien. Med. Wschr. **119** (1969), 785–787

Timonen, S., and *B. Meyer:* Correlation between Colposcopy, Cytology, and Histology, Ann. Chir. Gynaec. Fenn. **52** (1963), 338–350

Toger, A. E., and *E. V. Kokhanevich:* Microvascularisation of the Uterine Cervix in Intraepithelial and Invasive Cancer, Voprosy onkologii **19** (1973) 10, 3

Tosetti, K.: Methodik und Ergebnisse von kolposkopischen Reihenuntersuchungen (Methods and Results of Colposcopic Mass Screening). Dtsch. Gesundh. Wes. **10** (1955) 16, 580–582

Tovell, H. M. M., P. Banogan and *A. D. Nash:* Cytology and colposcopy in diagnosis and management of preclinical carcinoma of cervix uteri, Learning experience, Am. J. Obstet. Gynecol. **124** (1976) 8, 924

Treite, P.: Die Frühdiagnose des Plattenepithelkarzinoms am Collum uteri (Early Diagnosis of Squamous Cell Carcinoma of the Uterine Cervix). F. Enke Verlag, Stuttgart (1944)

Treite, P.: Zur Leistungsfähigkeit der Kolposkopie (Performance Potential of Colposcopy). Zbl. Gynäkol. (1942), 1458

Treite, P.: Leukoplakie und Karzinom (Leucoplakia and Carcinoma). Zbl. Gynäkol. (1952), 1570

Verschoof, K. J. H.: Über die Toluidinblauprobe in der kolposkopischen Diagnostik (Toluidine-Blue Test in Colposcopic Diagnosis). Mitt. Blatt Ges. Bekämpfg. Krebskrankh. Nordrhein-Westfalen, **5** (1969), 524 bis 525

Vetter, H.: Zur Frühdiagnose des Portiokarzinoms (Early Diagnosis of Portio Carcinoma). Gynaecologia (Basle) **134** Suppl. 2 (1957), 154–191

Vikshraitis, Ch. Ju., and *N. P. Motejunene:* Colposcopic Recognition of Cervical Precancer in Females Working with Certain Industrial Poisons, Voprosy onkologii **18** (1972) 12, 41

Volfson, N. T.: The Genesis of Glandlike Changes of Uterine Cervix, Neoplasma **20** (1973) 2, 189

Wagner, D., and *O. Fettig:* Zytologische und histologische Untersuchungen zur atypischen Umwandlungszone (Cytological and Histological Studies into Atypical Transformation Zone). Geburtsh. u. Frauenheilk. 1961

Walz, W.: Erfahrungsbericht über die Früherfassung des Portiokarzinoms unter besonderer Berücksichtigung der Kolpomikroskopie (Progress Report on Early Detection of Portio Carcinoma, with Particular Reference to Colpomicroscopy). Zschr. Geburtsh. Gynäkol. **144** (1955) 2, 117–154

Walz, W.: Früherfassung des Portiokarzinoms mit Hilfe der Kolposkopie, Zytologie und Kolpomikroskopie (Early Detection of Portio Carcinoma by means of Colposcopy, Cytology, and Colpomicroscopy) reviewed in Geburtsh. u. Frauenheilk. 15 (1955), 949

Walz, W.: Über die Genese der sogenannten indirekten Metaplasie im Bereich des Müllerschen Gang-Systems (Genesis of what is called Indirect Metaplasia in Müller's Duct System). Z. Geb. Gynäkol. 151 (1958), 1–21

Weiser, P.: Infrarotfotografie in der Gynäkologie (Infrared Photography in Gynaecology). Zbl. Gynäkol. 85 (1963), 1003–1008

Wespi, H. J.: Entstehung und Früherfassung des Portiokarzinoms (Genesis and Early Detection of Portio Carcinoma). Benno-Schwabe-Verlag, Basle (1946)

Wespi, H. J., and *W. Lotmar*: Fortschritte der Kolpofotografie und ihre Bedeutung (Progress in Colpophotography and Its Importance). Gynaecologia, Basle (1954), 5

Wespi, H. J.: Colpophotography, J. Biol. Photogr. Ass. 26 (1958), 59–68

Wespi, H. J.: What is the Place of Colposcopy in Modern Practice? J. Reproduct. Med. B. I. No. 1, 1968, Chicago, Lying-in Hospital

Wespi, H. J.: Die Rolle der Kolposkopie bei der Diagnose und beim Ausschluß des Zervixkarzinoms (Role of Colposcopy to Diagnose or Rule Out Cervical Carcinoma). Minerva Ginec. 22 (1970), 1148–1152

Wespi, H. J.: Stereokolpofotografie (Stereocolpophotography). Schweiz. Z. Gynäkol. Geburtsh. 2 (1971), 512–514

Wyss, H. J.: Zusammenhang zwischen kolposkopischen und histologischem Befund in der Schillerschen Abschabung (Correlations between Colposcopic and Histological Findings in Schiller's Scraping). Arch. Gyn. 194 (1961), 365–394

Youssef, A. F.: Colposcopy, J. Obstet. Gynaecol. of the British Empire

Zinser, H. K., and *G. Kern*: Kritische Betrachtungen zur Karzinomfrühdiagnostik (Critical Reflections on Early Diagnosis of Carcinoma). Geburtsh. u. Frauenheilk. 18 (1958) 2, 105–118

Zinser, H. K., and *K. H. Rosenbauer*: Untersuchungen an der gefäßinjizierten Cervix uteri (Studies into Uterine Cervix, following Vascular Injection) Geburtsh. u. Frauenheilk. 20 (1960), 658–660

Zinser, H. K.: Studien an der gefäßinjizierten Zervix (Studies into Cervix, following Vascular Injection). Geburtsh. u. Frauenheilk. 20 (1960), 651–657

Zinser, H. K., and *K. H. Rosenbauer*: Untersuchungen über die Angioarchitektonik der normalen und pathologisch veränderten Cervix uteri (Studies into Vascular Architecture of Normal and Pathologically Changed Uterine Cervix). Arch. Gynäkol. 194 (1960), 73–112

Zinser, H. L., *H. Meissner* and *H. P. Bötzelen*: Diagnostische und therapeutische Betrachtungen an 403 Frischfällen (Diagnostic and Therapeutic Observations on 403 New Cases). Geburtsh. u. Frauenheilk. 23 (1963) 4, 321–342

Zweifel, E.: Zur Frühdiagnose des Uteruskarzinoms durch Kolposkopie (Early Diagnosis of Uterus Carcinoma by means of Colposcopy). Münch. med. Wschr. (1933), 1145

Subject index

Plates

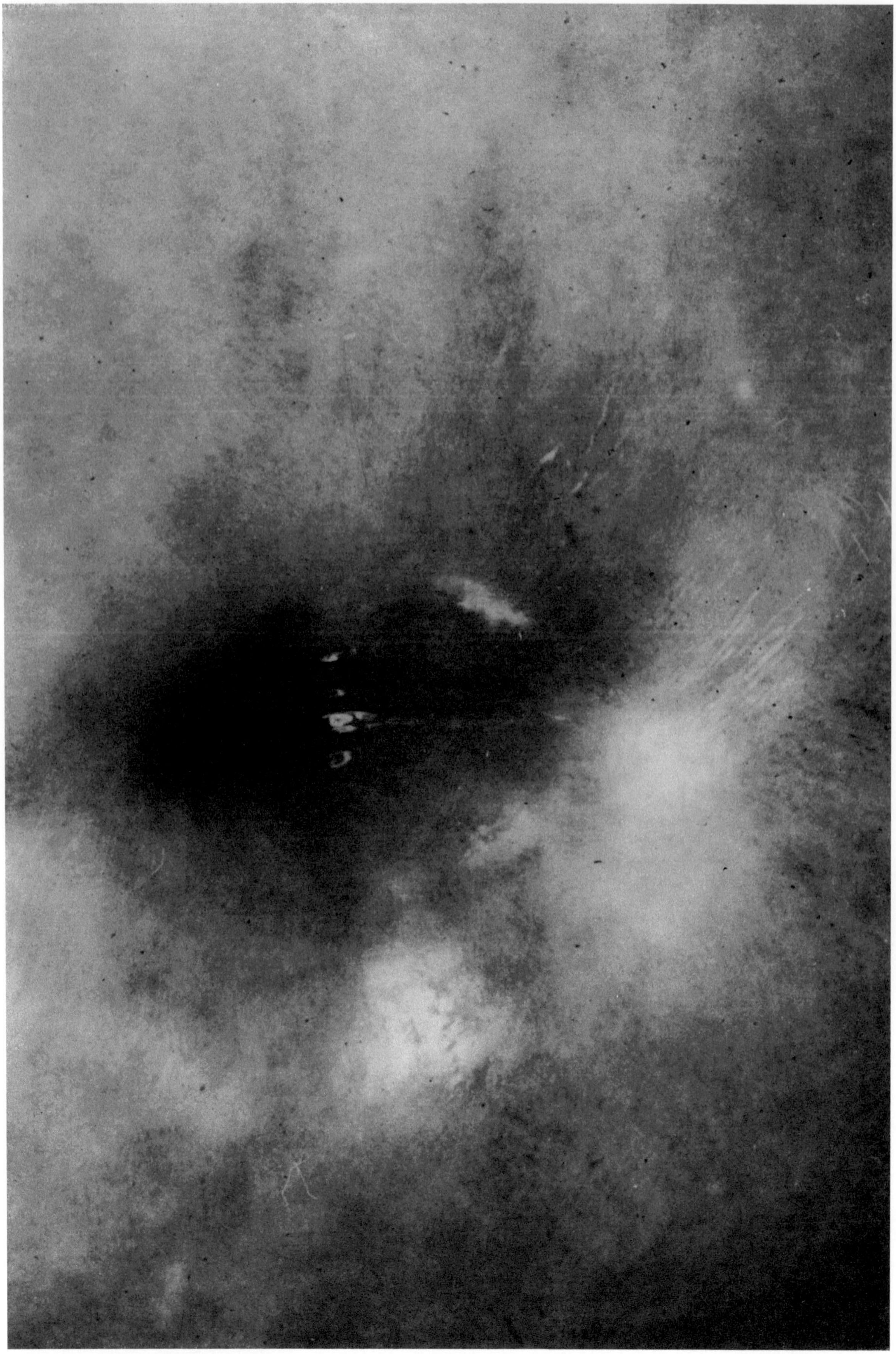

Plate 1 **Original squamous epithelium**

Original portio in early menopause with squamous epithelium thinned, smooth surface and normal network capillaries, absence of stronger vessels, pitted os uteri, clear cervical mucus.

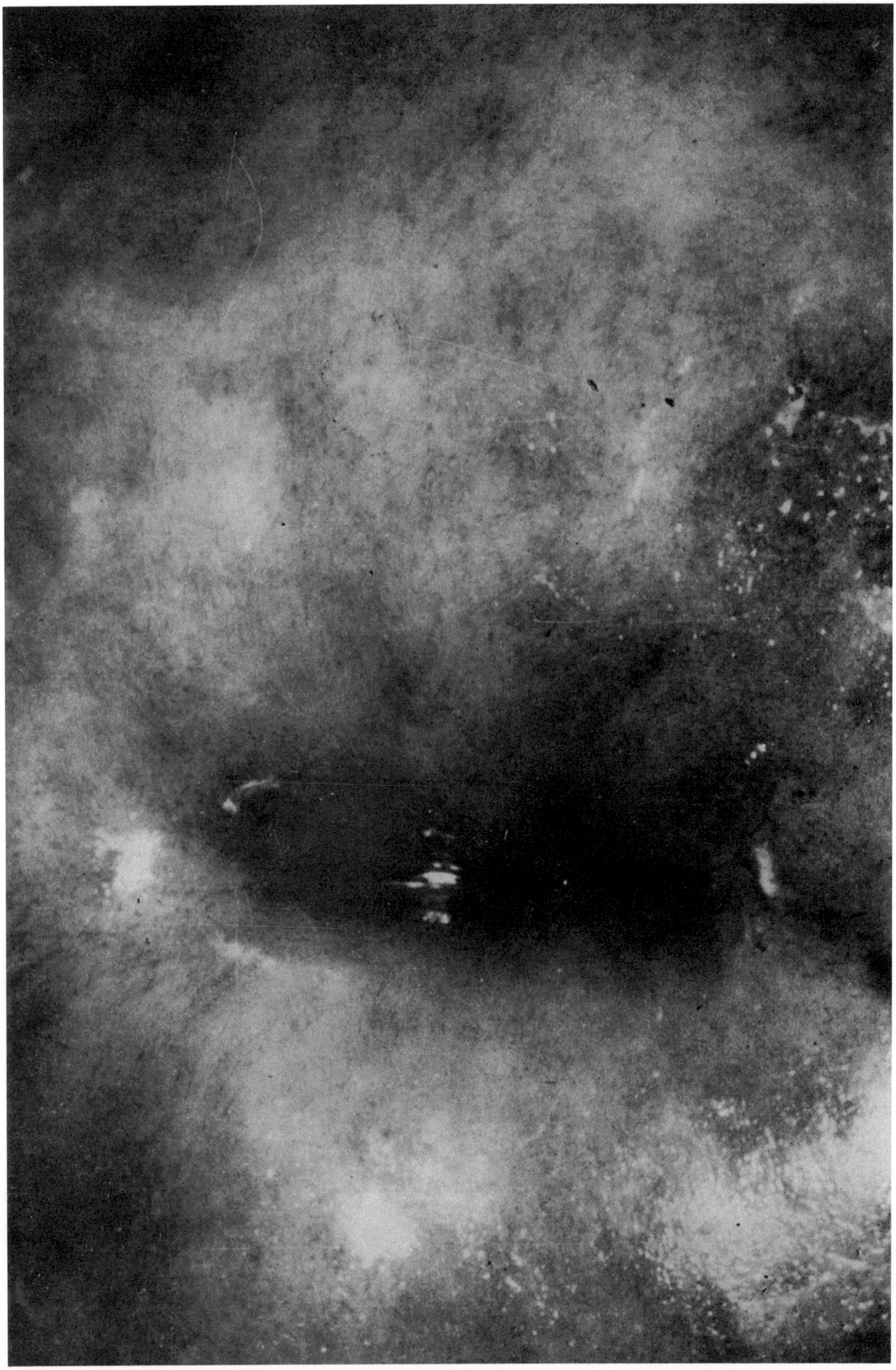

Plate 2 Original squamous epithelium

Ideal clinical picture of original portio of woman in sexual maturity, squamous epithelium in normal stratification, surface relief granulated, normal vessels of hairpin and network types, reflecting surface, clear cervical mucus.

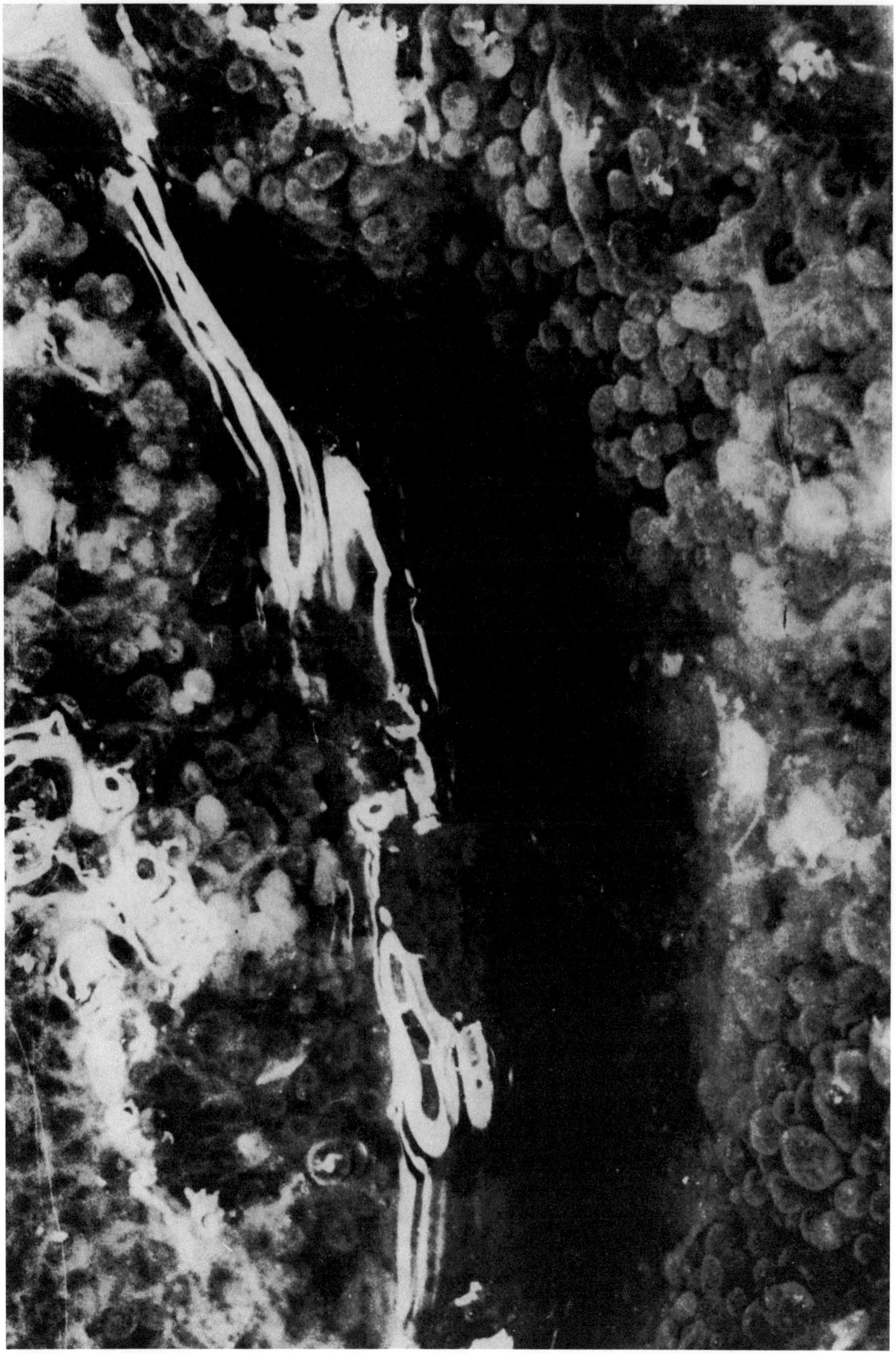

Plate 3 Columnar epithelium

Papillary to villous ectopy, following application of acetic acid in concentration of three per cent, extending from endocervical canal to portio, excessive secretion of mucus in responce to hormonal contraceptives.

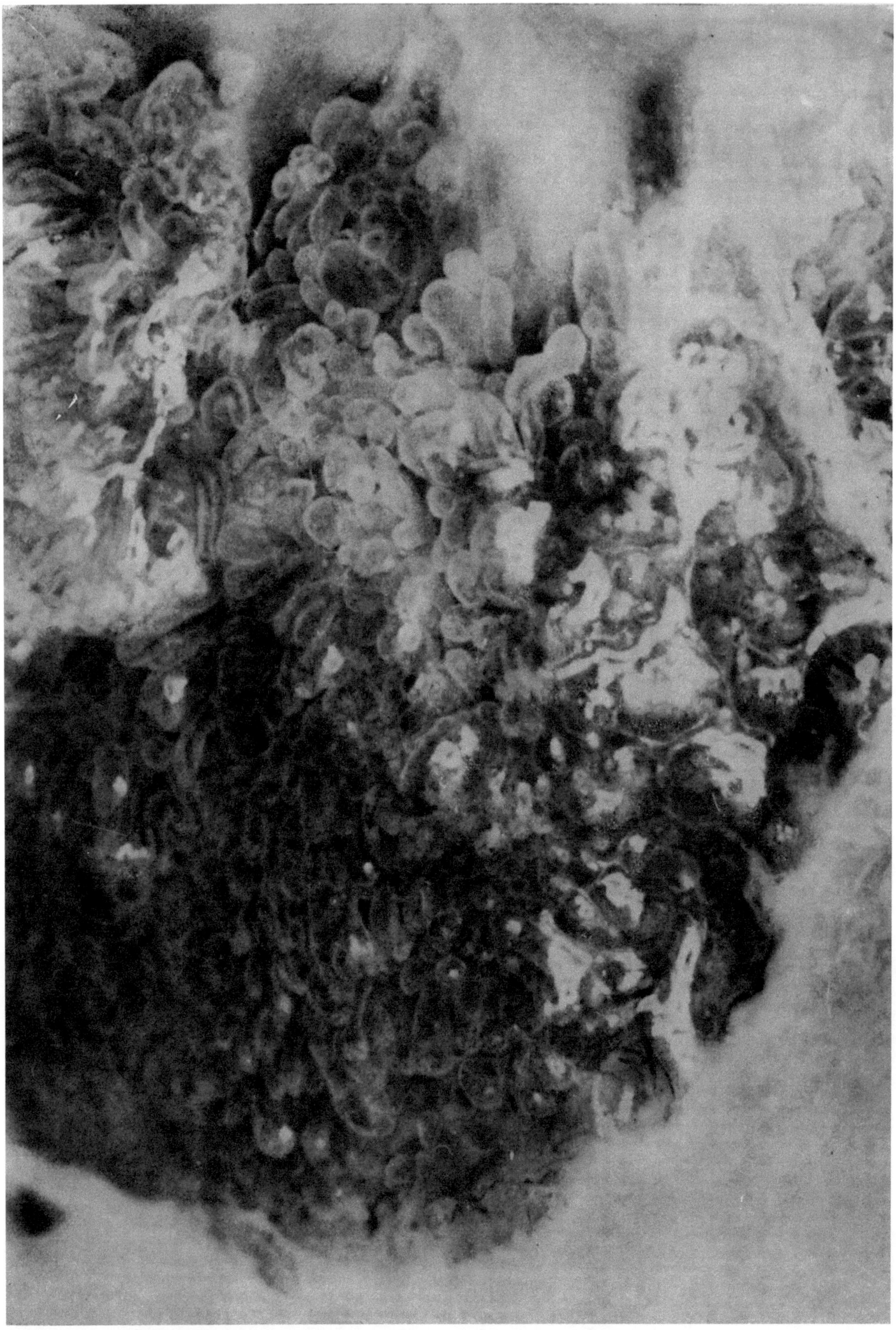

Plate 4 Columnar epithelium

Papillary ectopy, following application of acetic acid in concentration of three per cent, distinct delimitation from squamous epithelium, visibility of vessels in boundary areas gradually restored along with declining action of acetic acid.

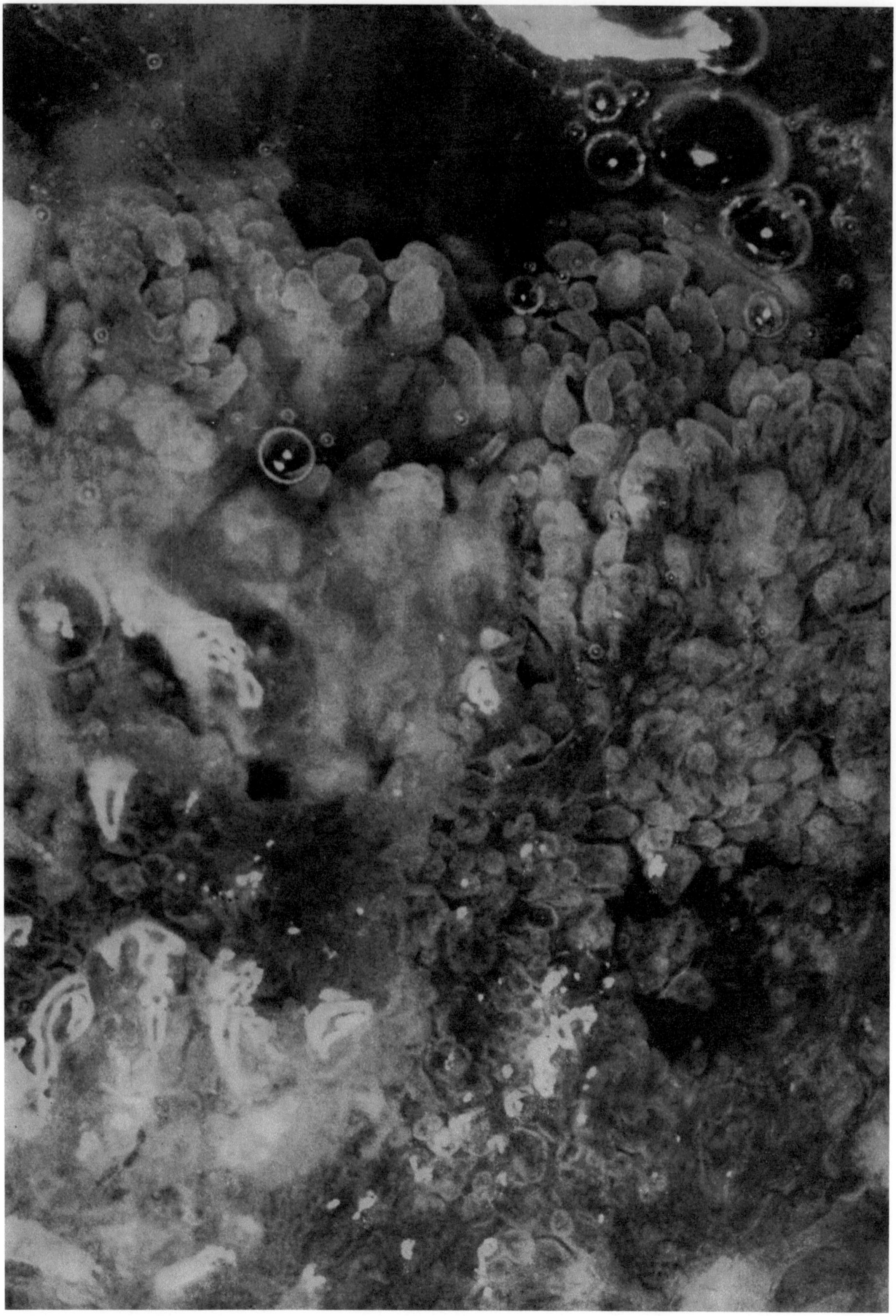

Plate 5 Columnar epithelium

Polypous ectopy accompanied by signs of inflammation in early gravidity, strong vascularisation, use of acetic acid followed by hypersecretion of somewhat turbid mucus.

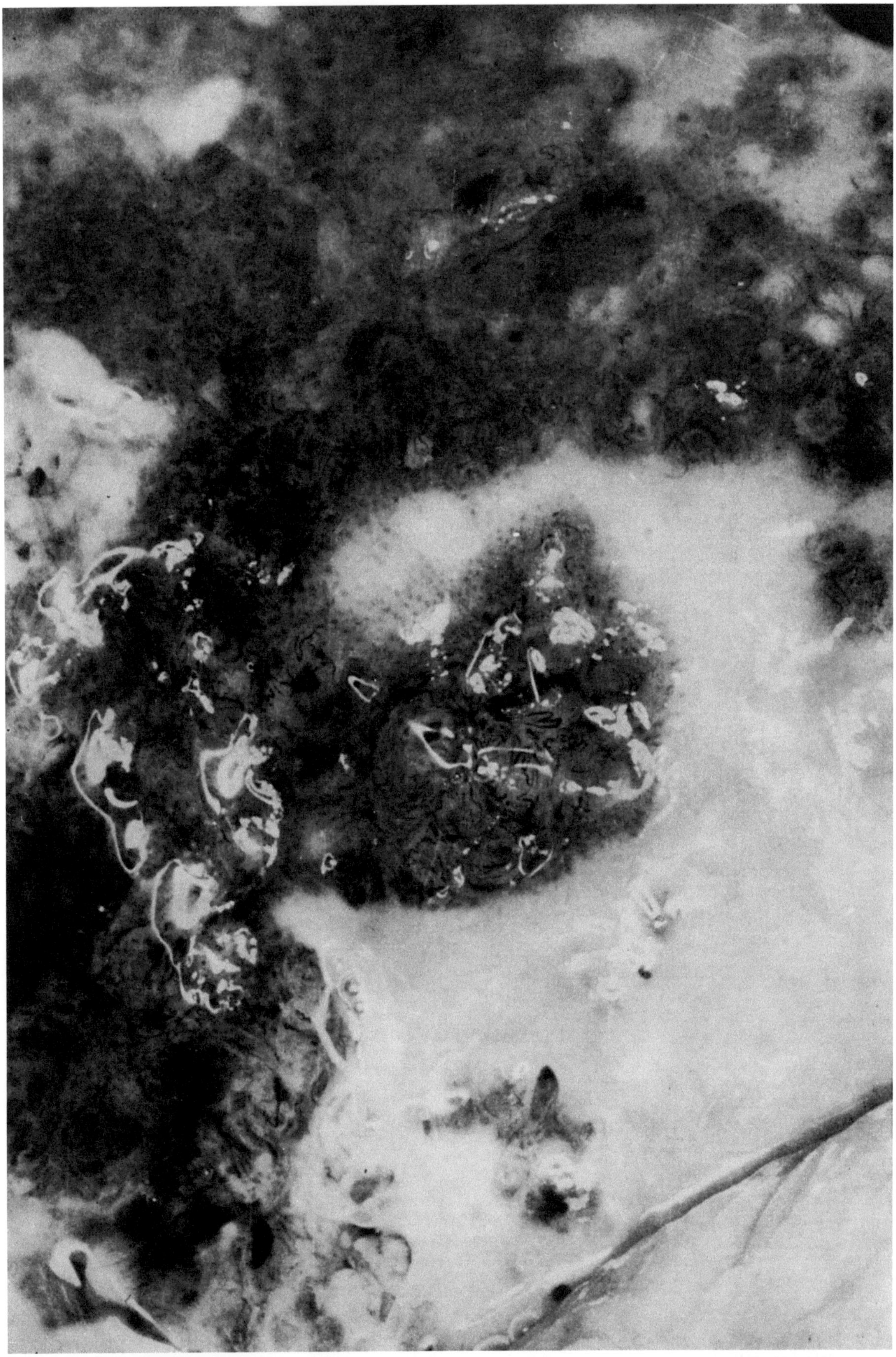

Plate 6 Columnar epithelium and transformation zone

Ectopic columnar epithelium with areas of incipient metaplastic transformation, without use of acetic acid; can be easily confused macroscopically and colposcopically with carcinoma, since impression of neoplastic vessels, comparable to atypical hairpin capillaries, can be easily created by superimposed inflammation; use of acetic acid, therefore, necessary for colposcopy.

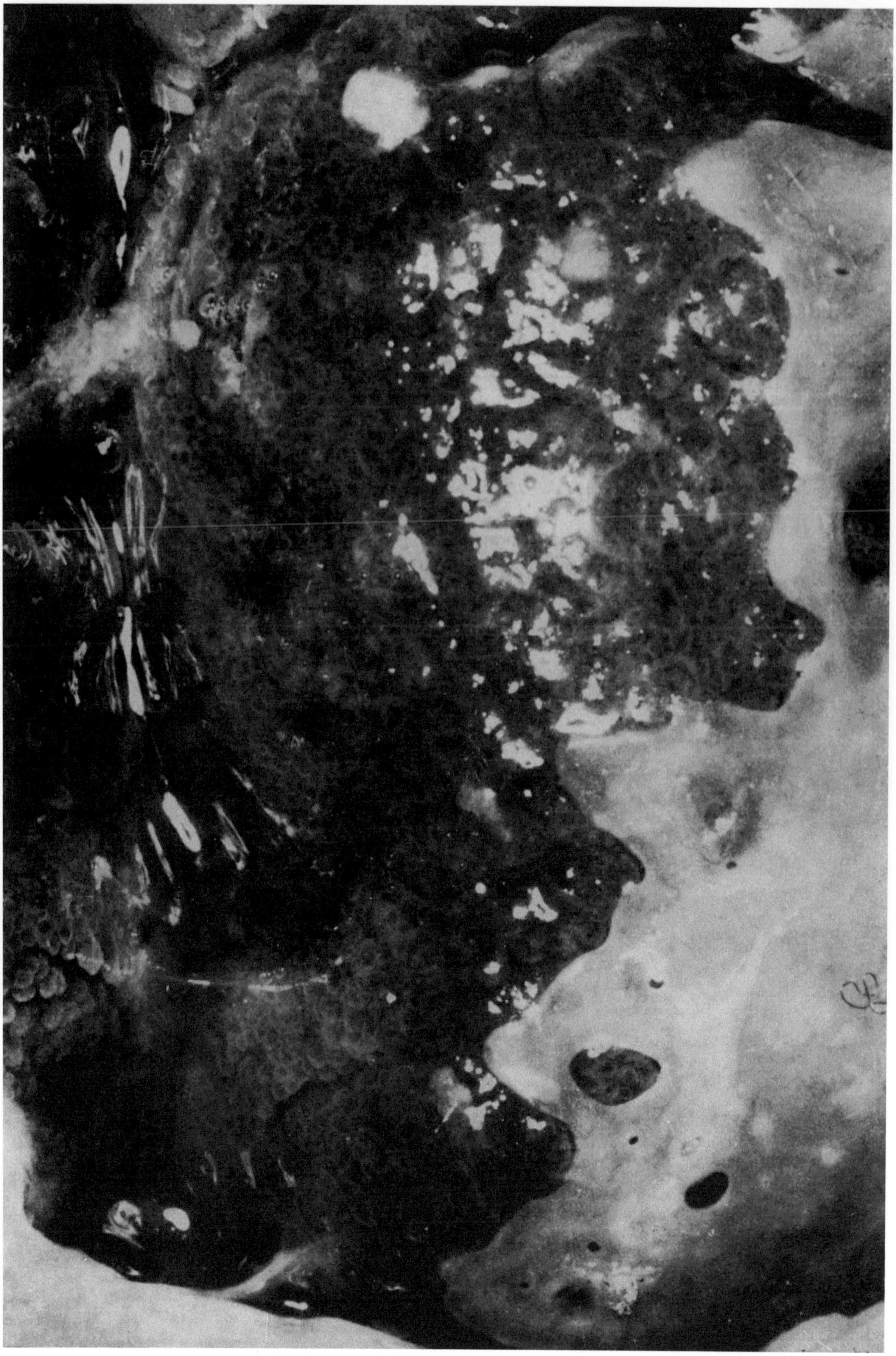

Plate 7 Columnar epithelium and transformation zone

Use of acetic acid followed by appearance on portio surface of small round grapes, colposcopic reflection of deformation of uterine cervix in terms of ectropionisation, depending on ovarian function of woman; vessels beneath columnar epithelium are no longer visible, following application of acetic acid, but neoplastic vessels are; metaplastic squamous epithelium, located flush with original epithelium and stained white in response to acetic acid, penetrating from margin of ectopy.

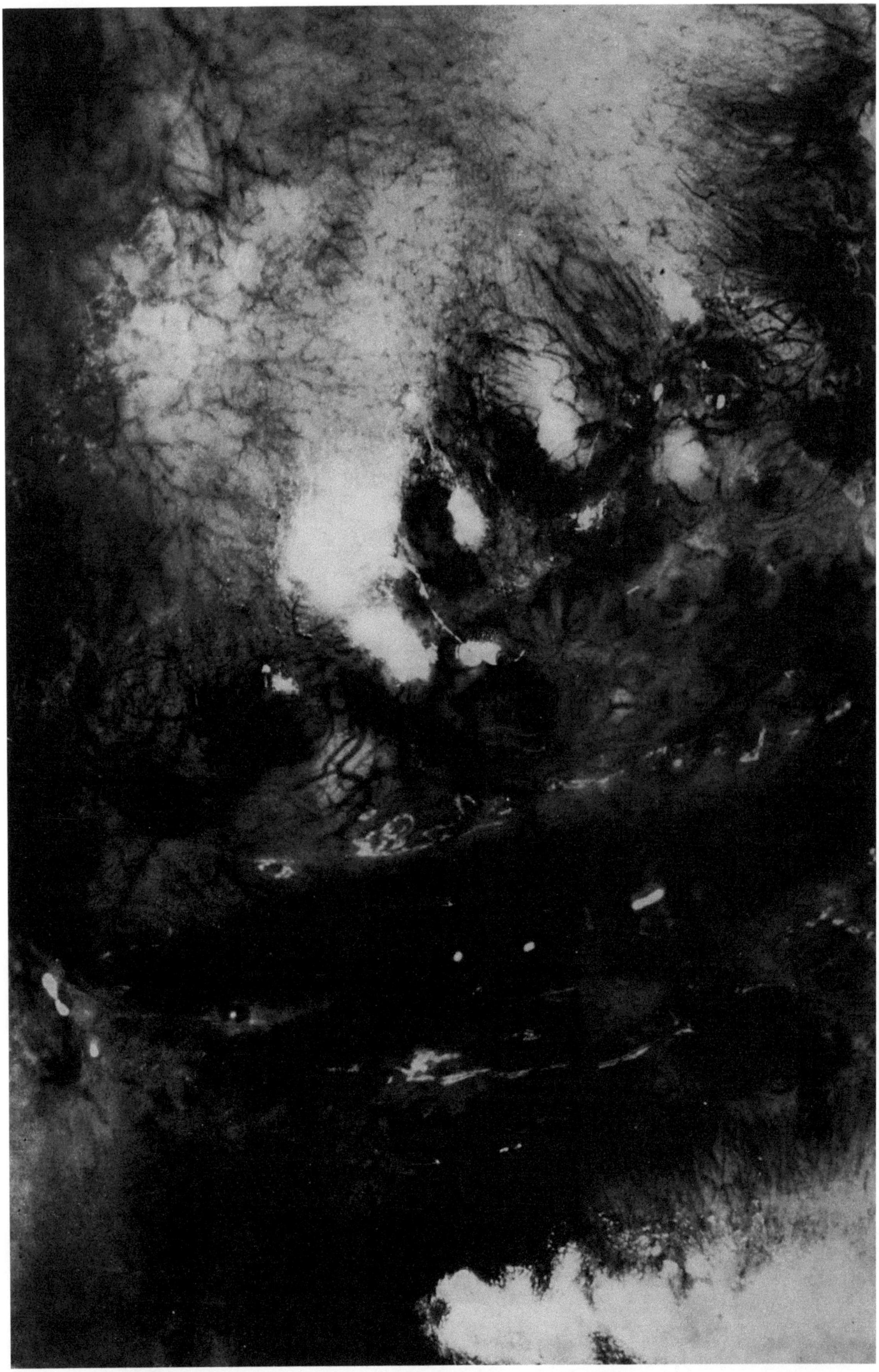

Plate 8 **Transformation zone**

With open transformation zone, squamous epithelium again present on portio but not comparable with squamous epithelium of original portio; being some sort of "membrane suis generis", its biological position lies between original squamous epithelium and columnar epithelium of ectopy; colourful colposcopic picture of transformation zone characterised by "glands" within squamous epithelium as residence of columnar epithelium which had been ectopic before; vessels of transformation zone ramified like branches, clusters or twigs; normal ramification vessels and "glands" being criteria of transformation zone.

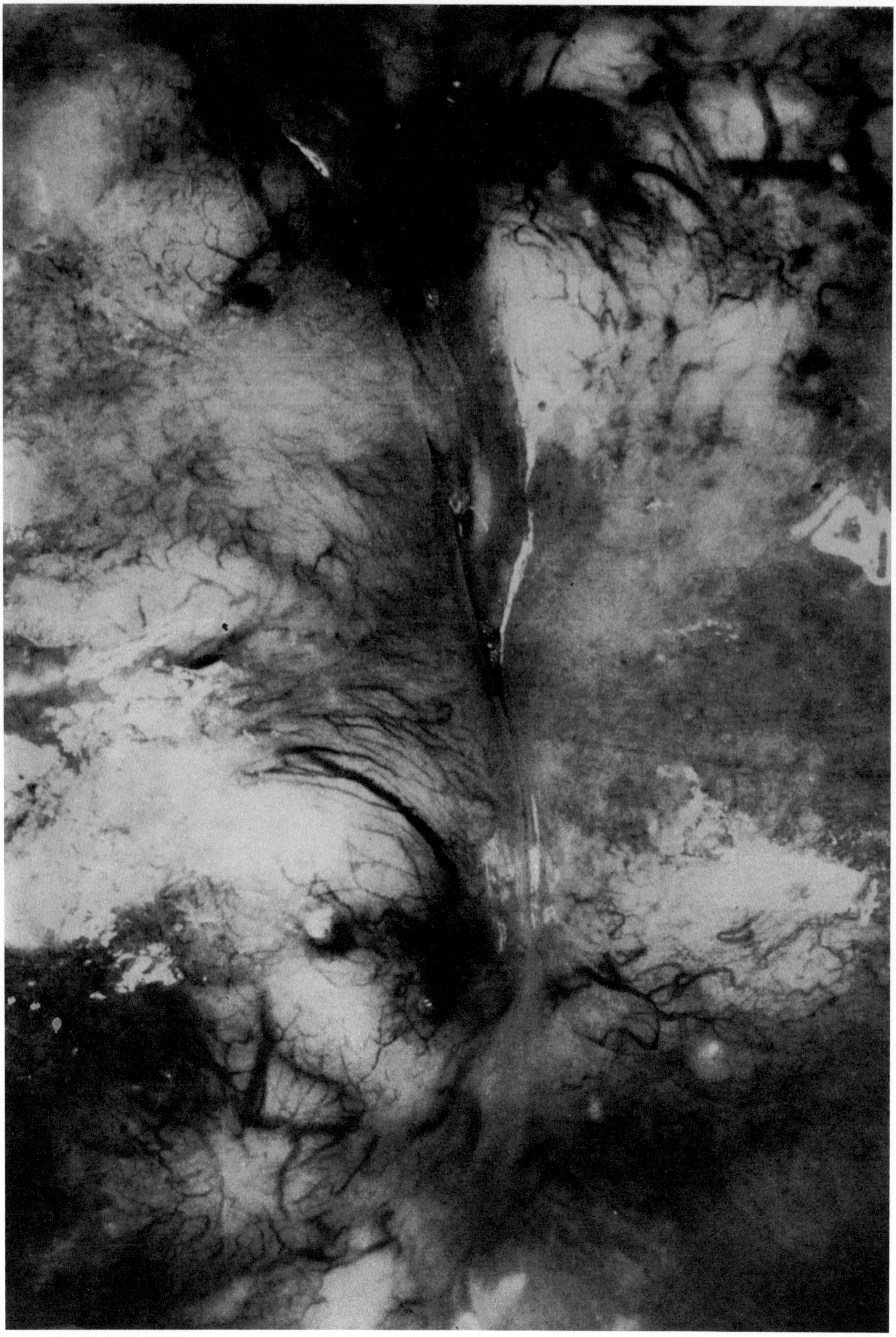

Plate 9 **Transformation zone**

Closed transformation zone; processes of epidermisation completed; glandular openings no longer visible, but small and big retention cysts are, with typical vascular pattern of transformation zone being clearly recognisable above them; vessels in genuinely dichotomous ramification with continuously declining diameter; varicose vessels rarely detectable; possibility of pulsatory stenosis and dilatation of vessels.

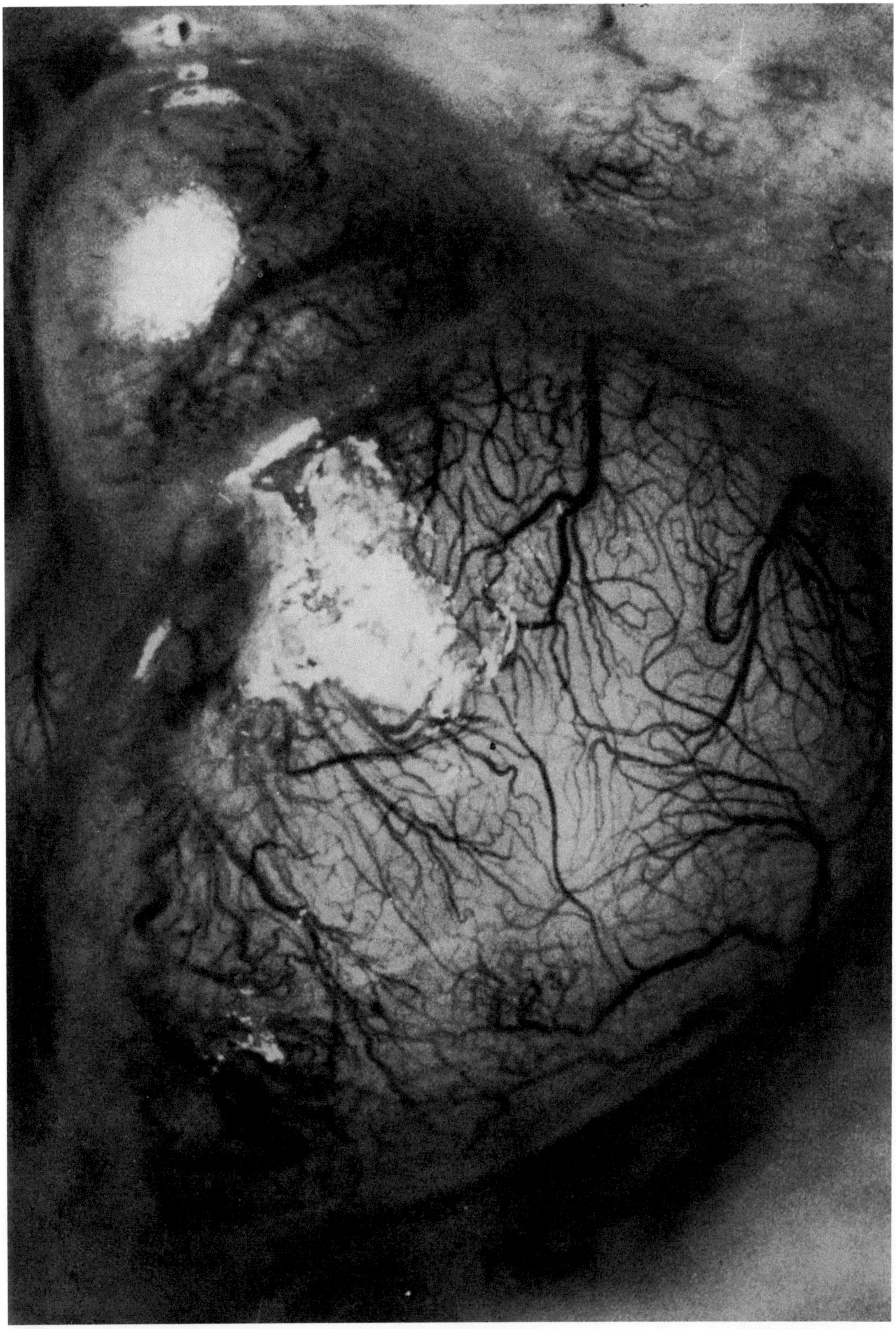

Plate 10 Transformation zone

Naboth's ovules are large retention cysts; typical, normally ramified vessels of transformation zone clearly visible; these vessels may be in crosswise overlapping, a pattern explainable by their origin and development; general regularity of vascular pattern.

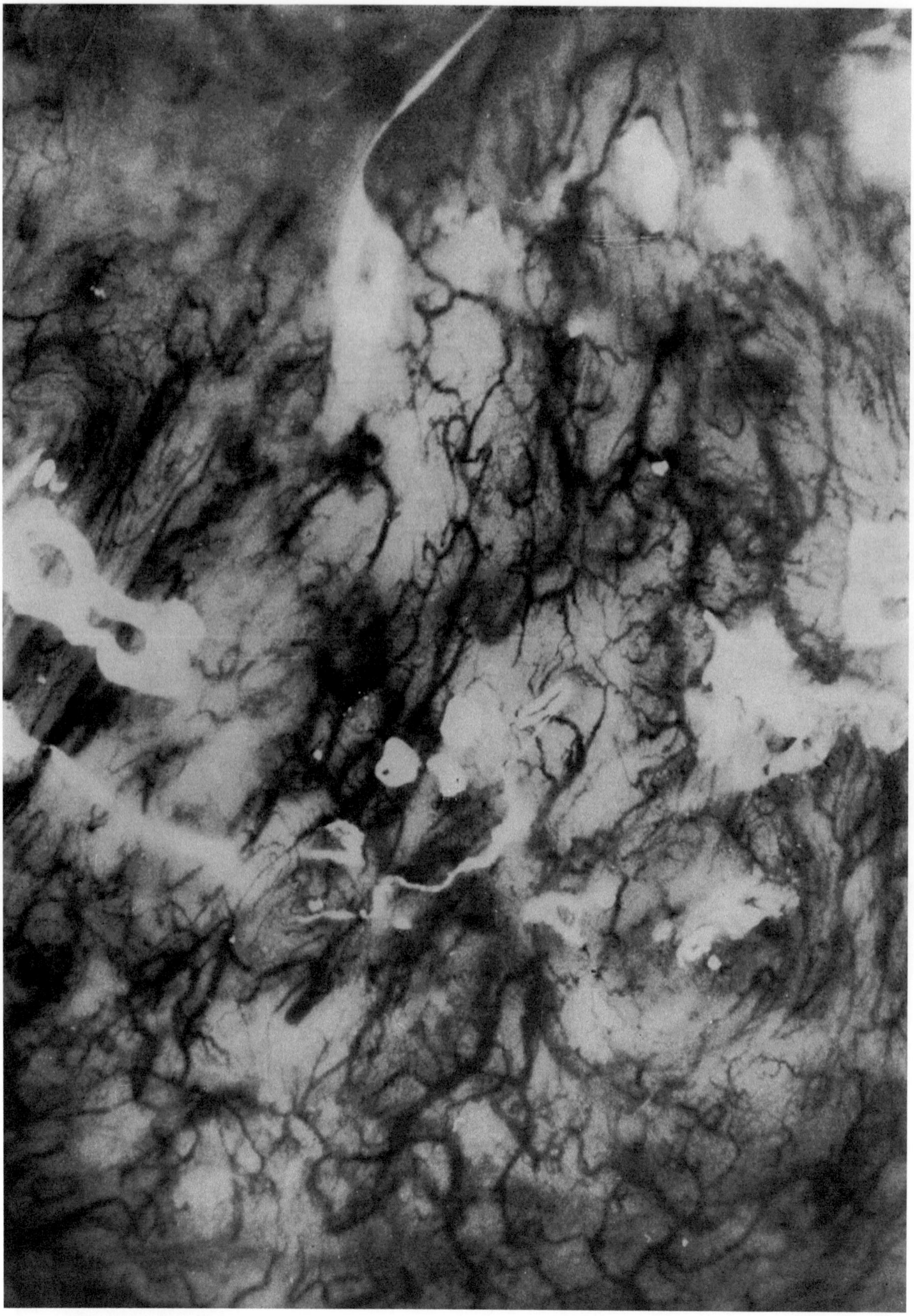

Plate 11 Transformation zone

Highly vascularised transformation zone often with vessels of ramification and network types; recordable from thin metaplastic squamous epithelium with possibility for terminal vessels to shine through.

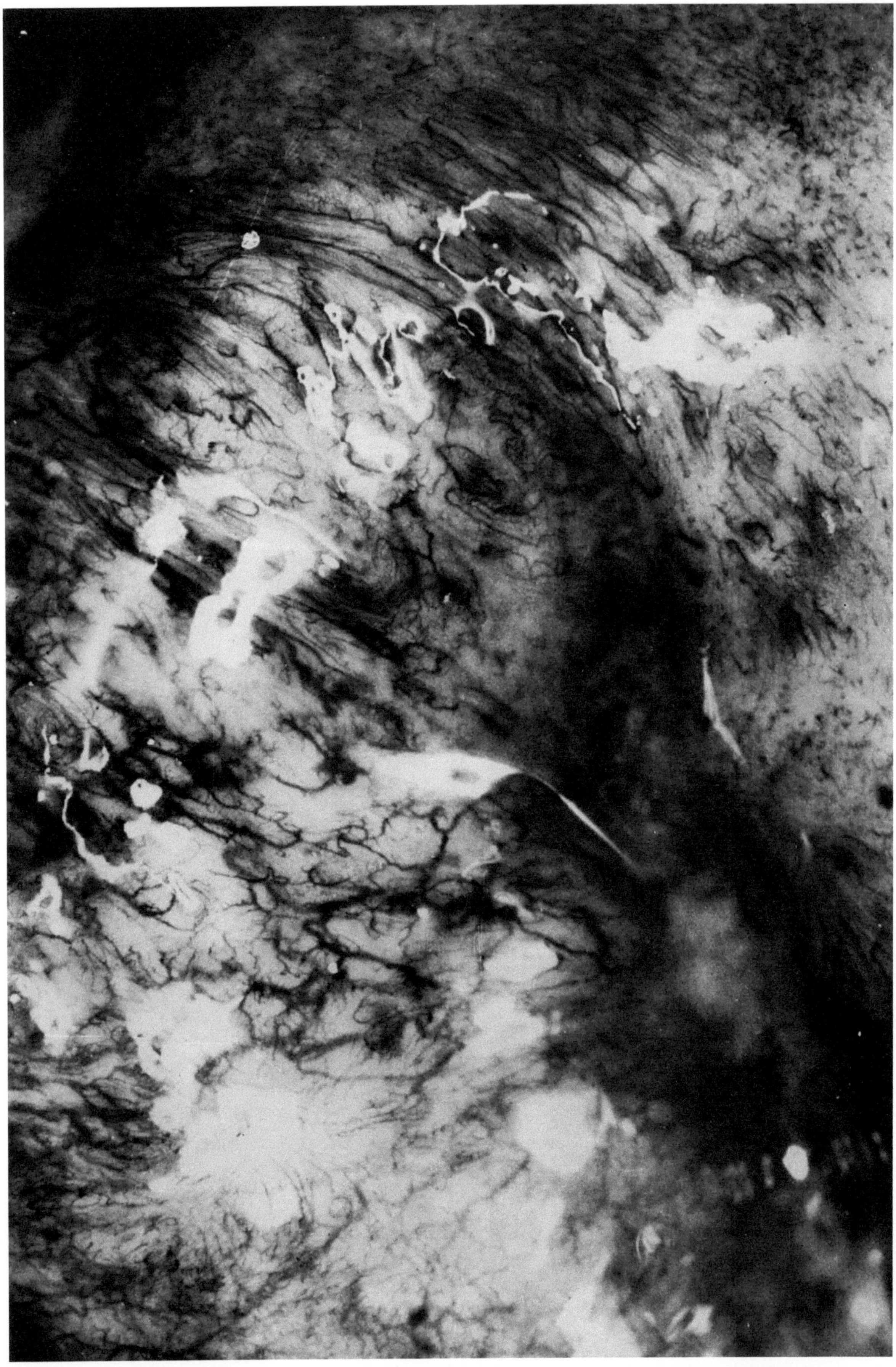

Plate 12 Transformation zone

Highly vascularised transformation zone with numerous long-drawn but normally subdivided vessels; also visible are vessels of normal network and hairpin types.

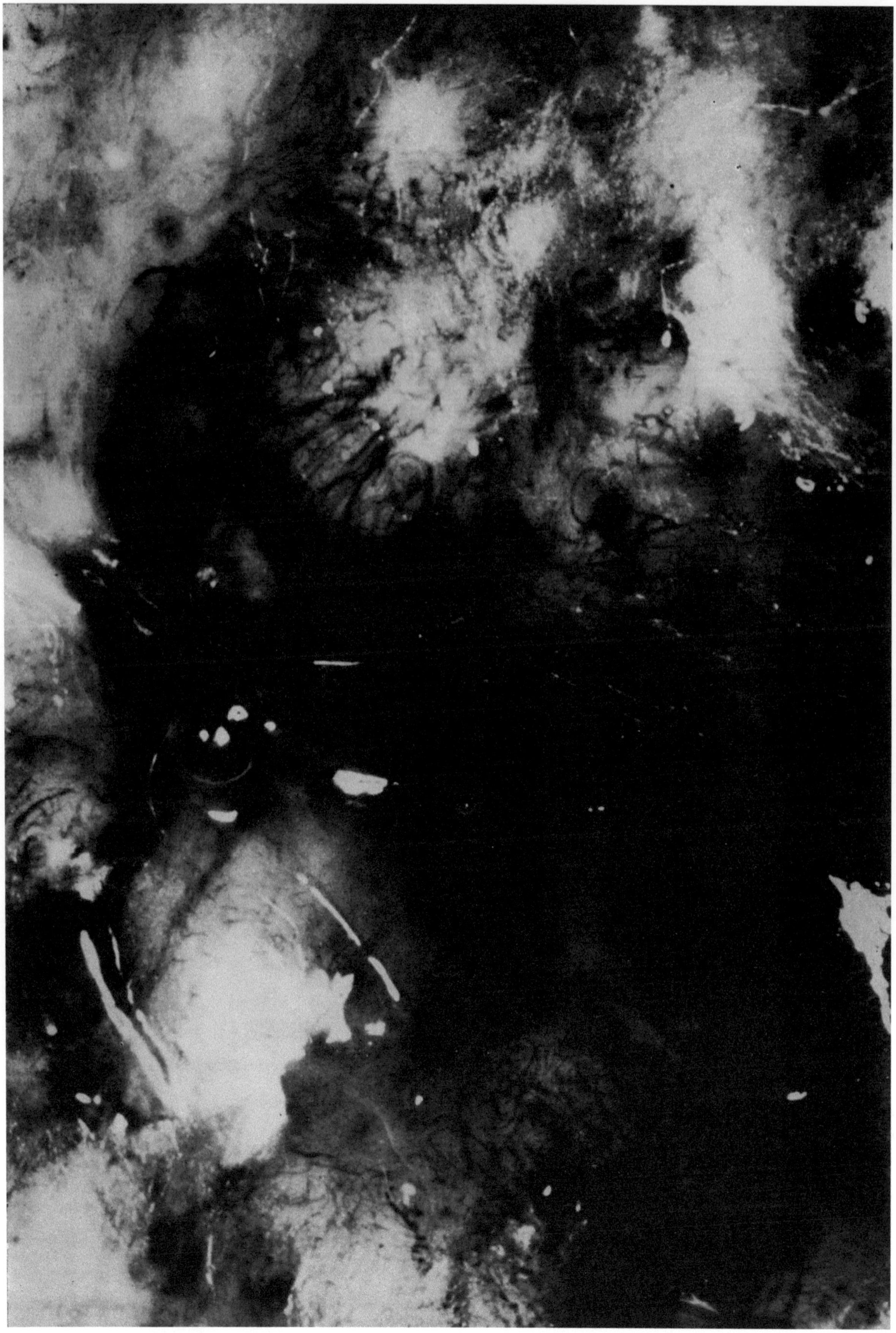

Plate 13 **Transformation Zone**

Large-calibre, rapidly ramifying vessels shooting from margin into epidermisation area of highly vascularised transformation zone; vessels of network type interspersed; high vascularisation of transformation zone reflects high rate of regeneration and, therefore, should be followed up carefully by means of colposcopic and cytological procedures, for the purpose of earliest dossible detection of any pathological regeneration.

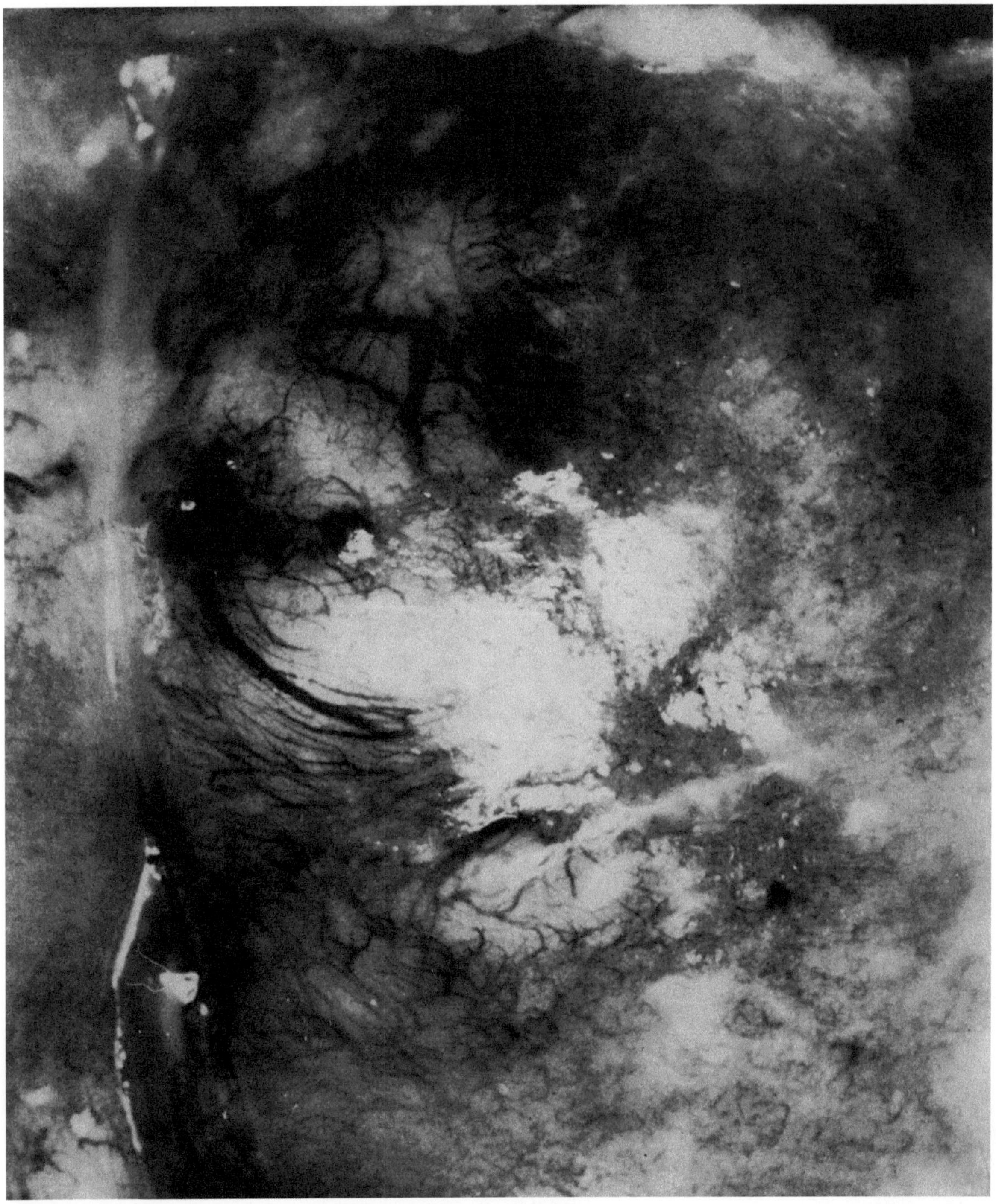

Plate 14 Transformation zone
Residual large-calibre vessels of old close transformation zone.

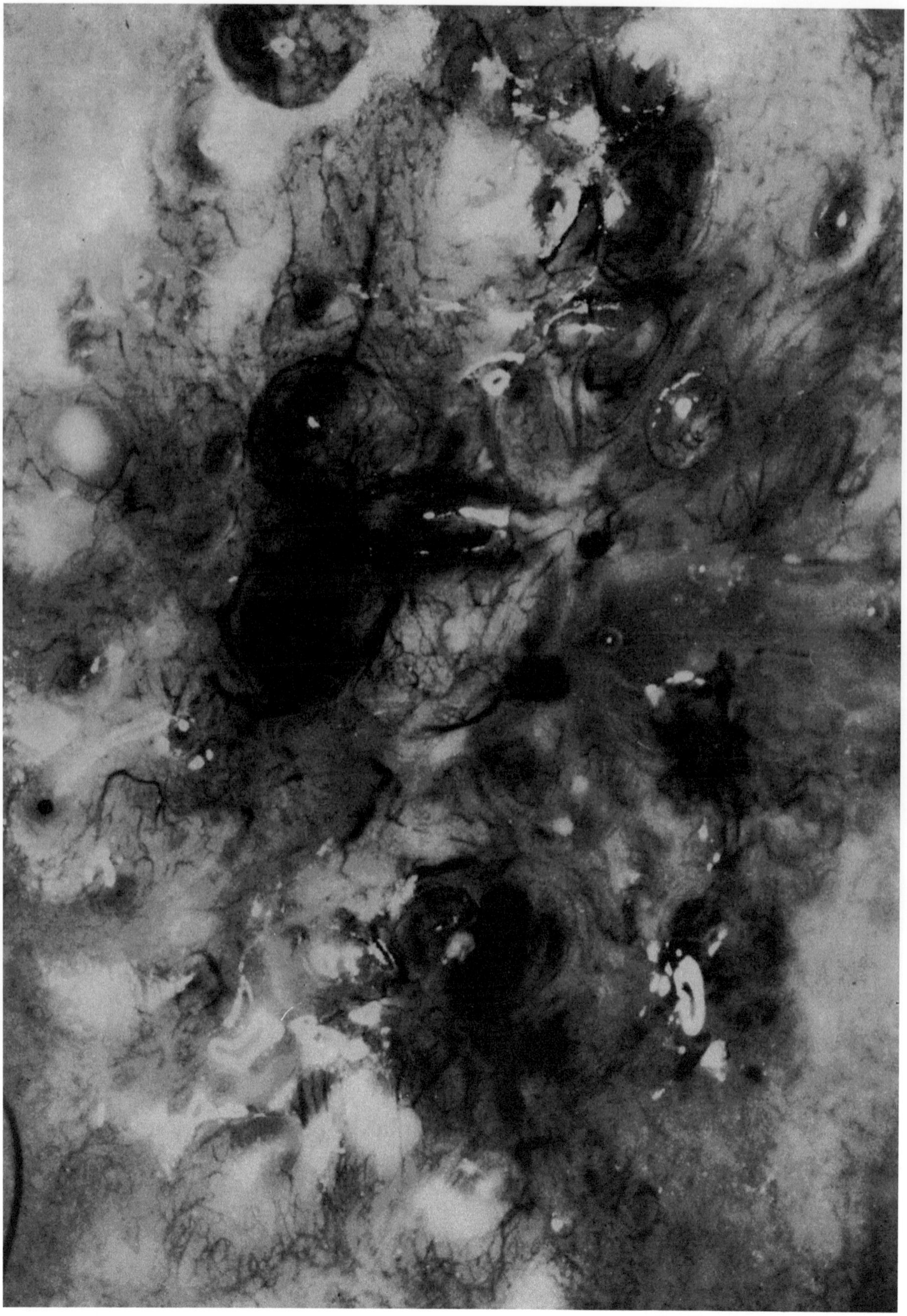

Plate 15 Vascular atypia

Vascular atypia occurs quite often in a transformation zone atypical by delimited definition; compilation of findings which may cause problems of interpretation even to the experienced examiner and are usually grouped by vascular atypias (suspicious transformation zone and abnormal transformation zone are synonyms); particular attention required in any case; findings include plenty of vascularisation with vessels in irregular positions, disruption and variation of calibres, whitish-keratinised glandular openings, vessels in circular arrangement around glandular openings, as well as apparently avascular areas and trend to keratinisation.

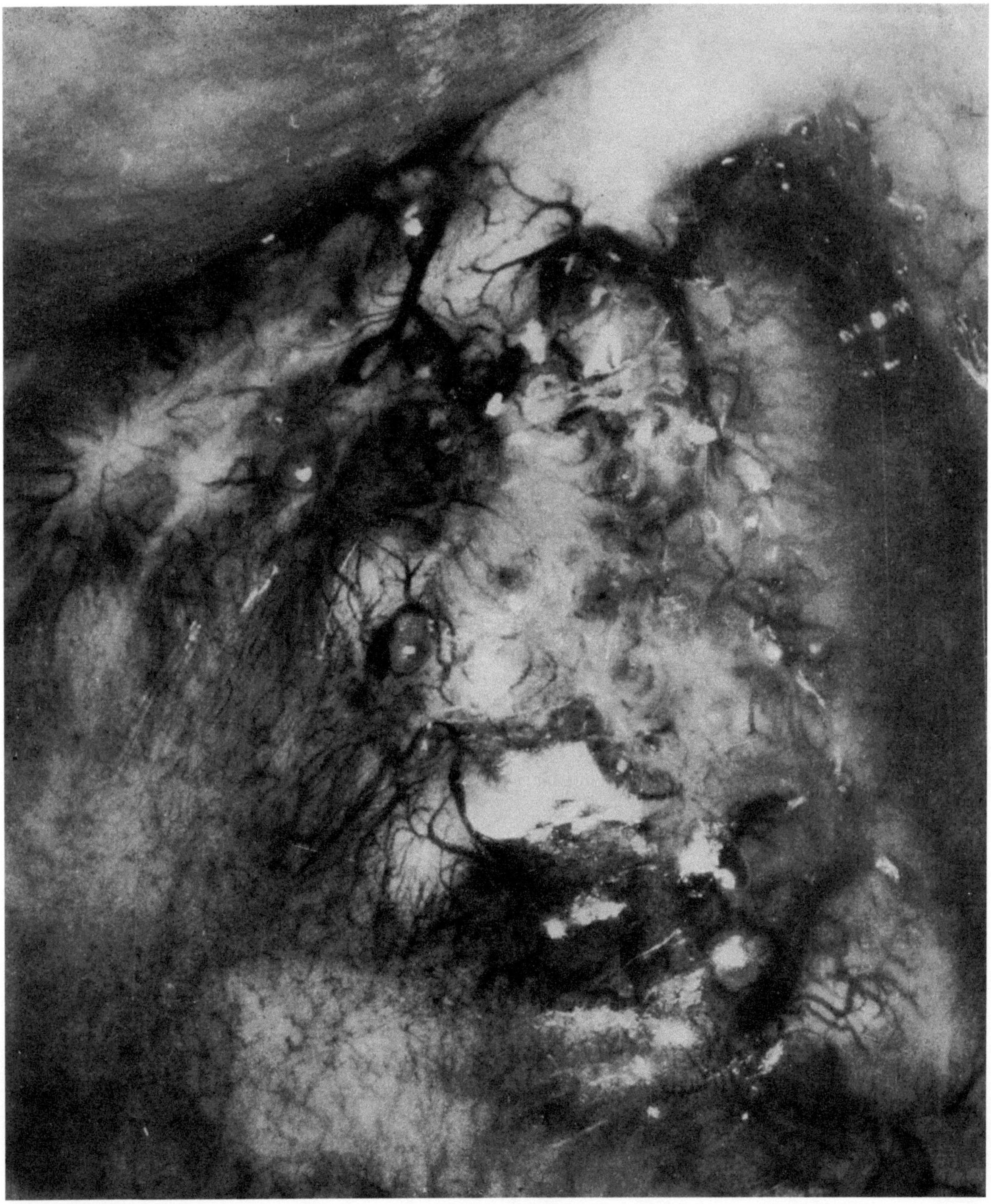

Plate 16 **Vascular atypia**

Vessels in normal arborisation, open glands, and small retention cysts accompanied by atypical vessel disruptures, visible at upper margin of Plate.

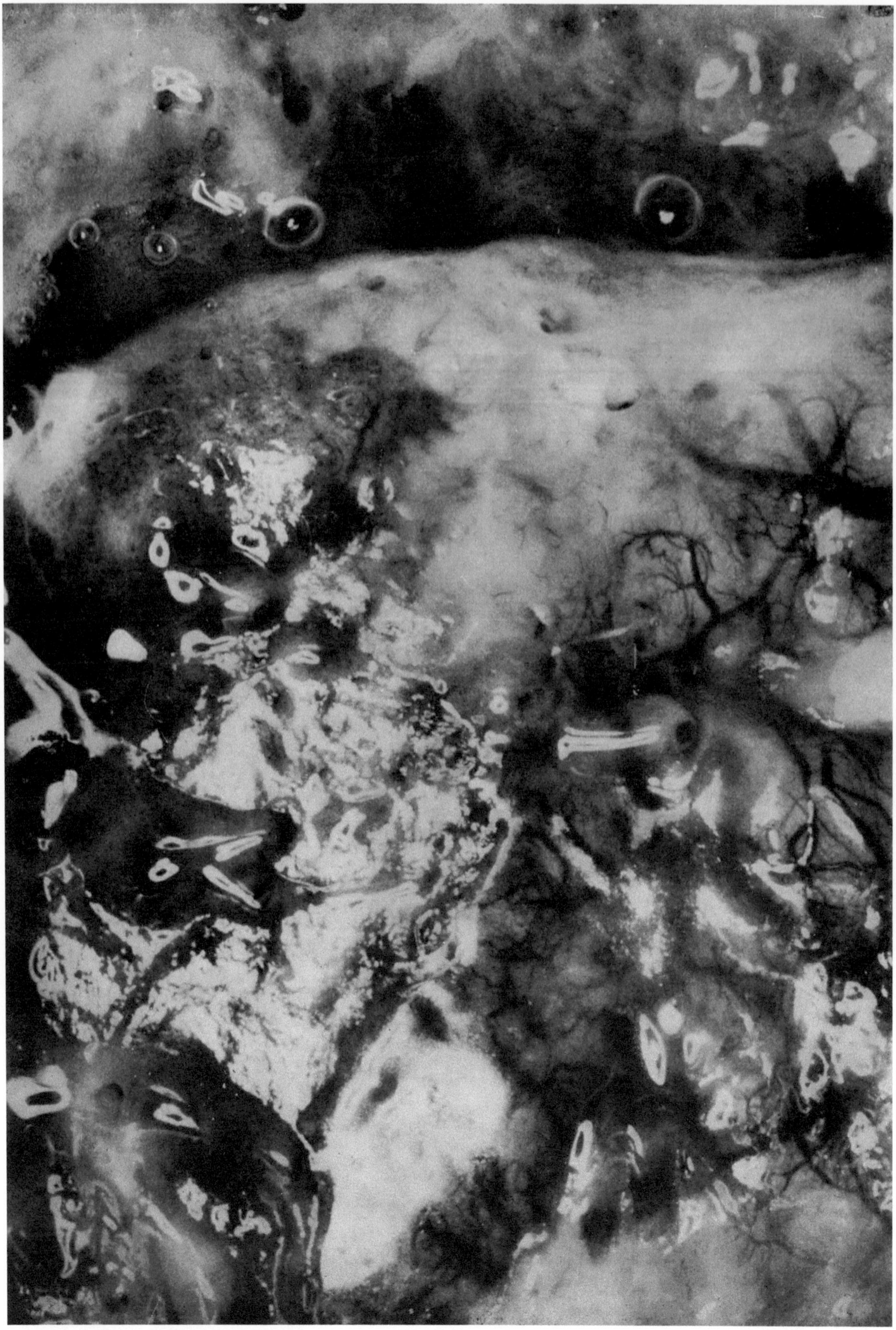

Plate 17 Vascular atypia and keratosis

Typically regular subdivision and arrangement of vessels in visible coexistence with strongly meandering vessels, atypical hairpin capillaries, and comma-shaped vessels with whitish opaque hyperplastic epithelia, some of them keratotic; glandular openings warped and keratinised; conspicuous difference in levels; early invasive carcinoma histologically secured.

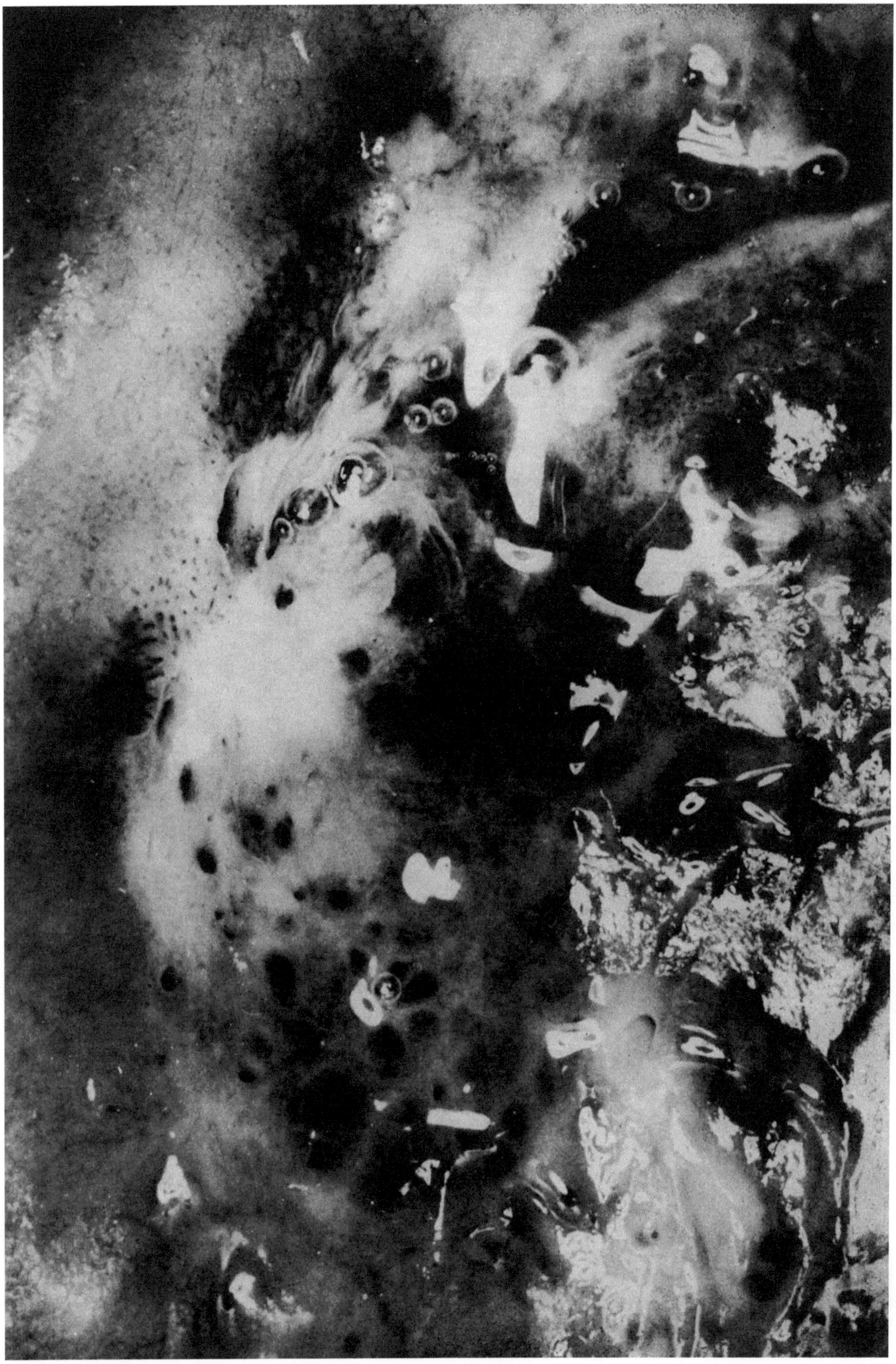

Plate 18 **Keratosis, punctuation, and mosaic**
Keratinised glandular openings, white epithelium without transparency, many small papillae with cork-screw capillaries, atypical hairpin capillaries, and negative field pattern.

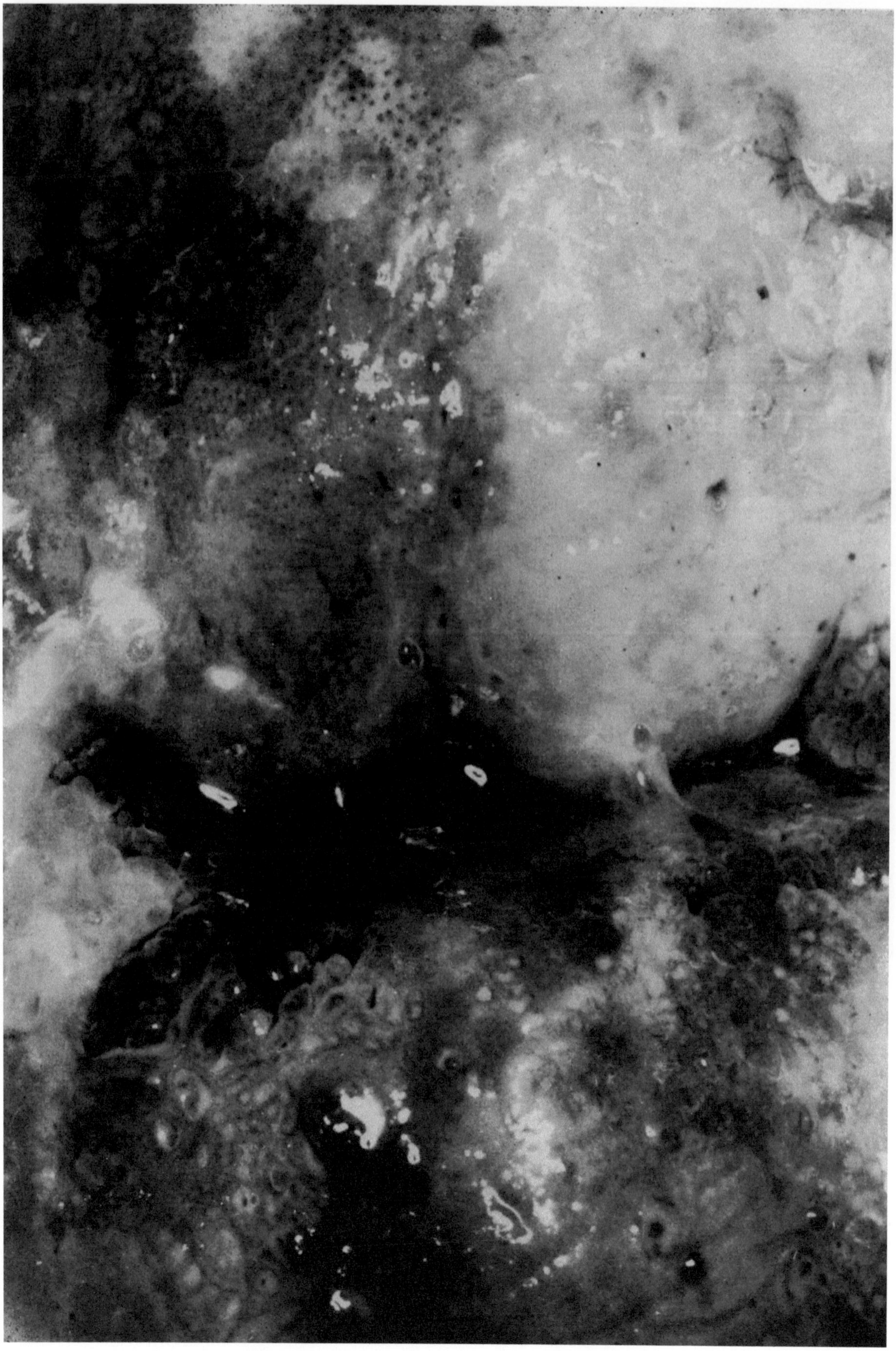

Plate 19 Columnar epithelium, transformation zone, mosaic, punctuation, and keratosis

Normal findings may be accompanied by abnormal colposcopic pictures, if ectopic columnar epithelium is replaced by pathologically transformed squamous epithelium: area of posteroir labium of os uteri exhibits normal columnar epithelium in juvenile transformation zone and, next to it, glandular openings, some with white rims, others with warped walls; anterior labium of os uteri shows field pattern areas, simple and papillary floor, as well as leucoplakially thickened metaplastic squamous epithelium.

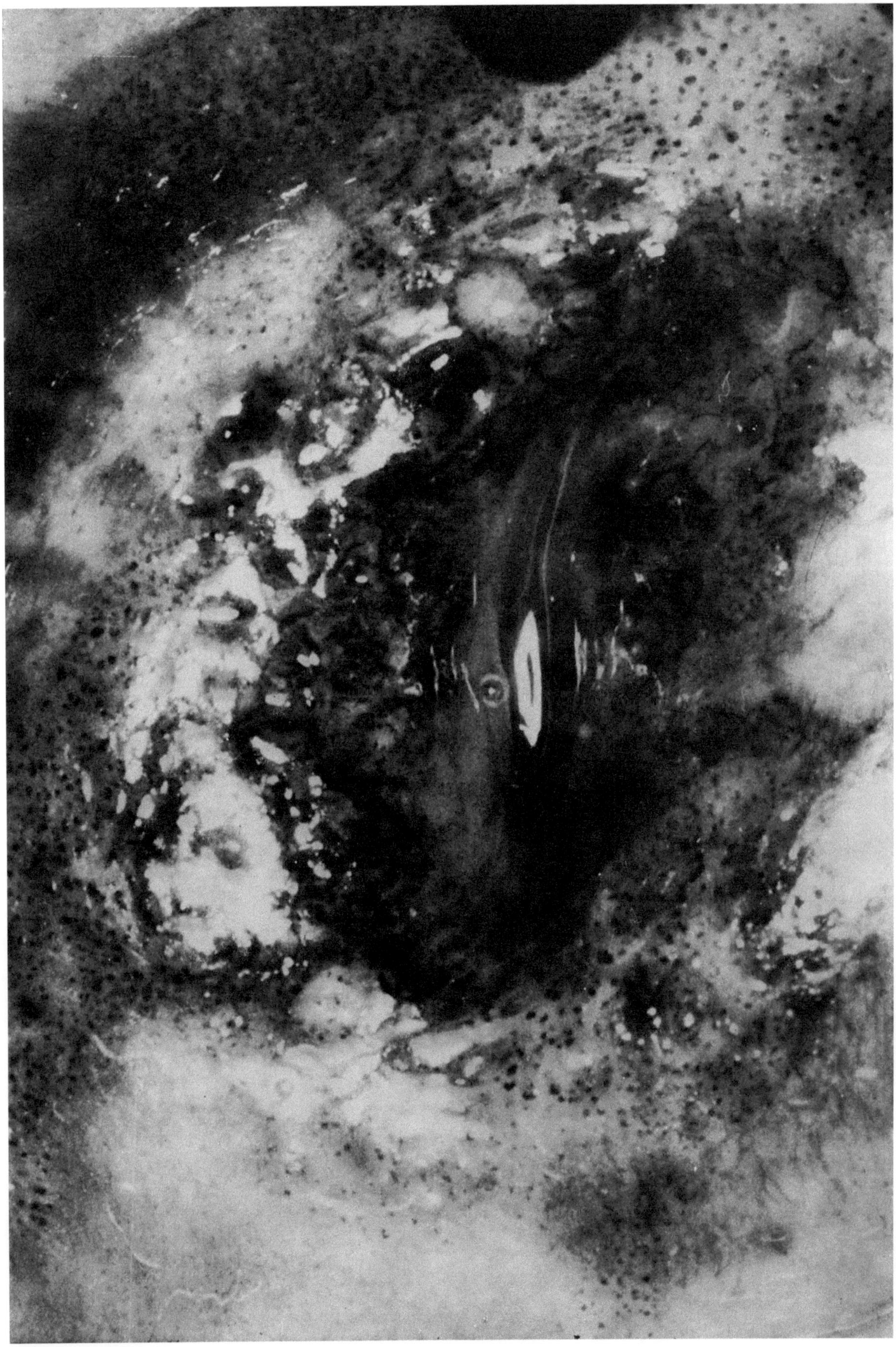

Plate 20 Punctuation

While *Hinselmann's* definition of basic regions was to mean leucoplakia areas which had temporarily lost their coating layers, the same findings, today, are summarised under a cover term which has to satisfy the following criteria: distinctly delimited, colourfully conspicuous areas in which atypical hairpin capillaries are visible; interpreted as tender, simple, and papillary floor, depending on vascular spacings and atypia.

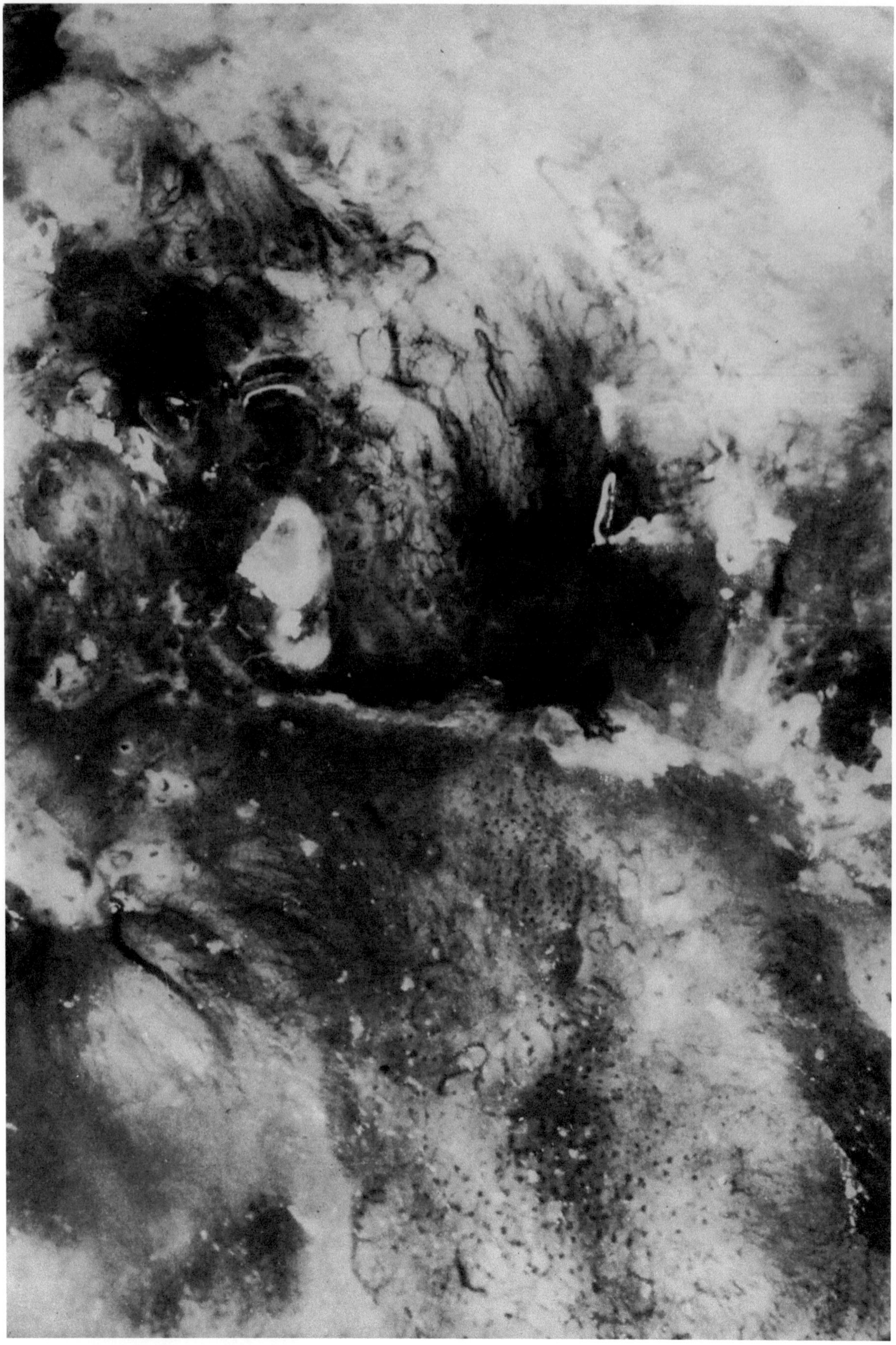

Plate 21 **Punctuation, mosaic, invasive carcinoma**

Simple papillary floor, with field pattern structures slightly indicated at posterior labium of os uteri; typically washed-out picture of carcinoma with pertinent vessels detectable from anterior labium of os uteri.

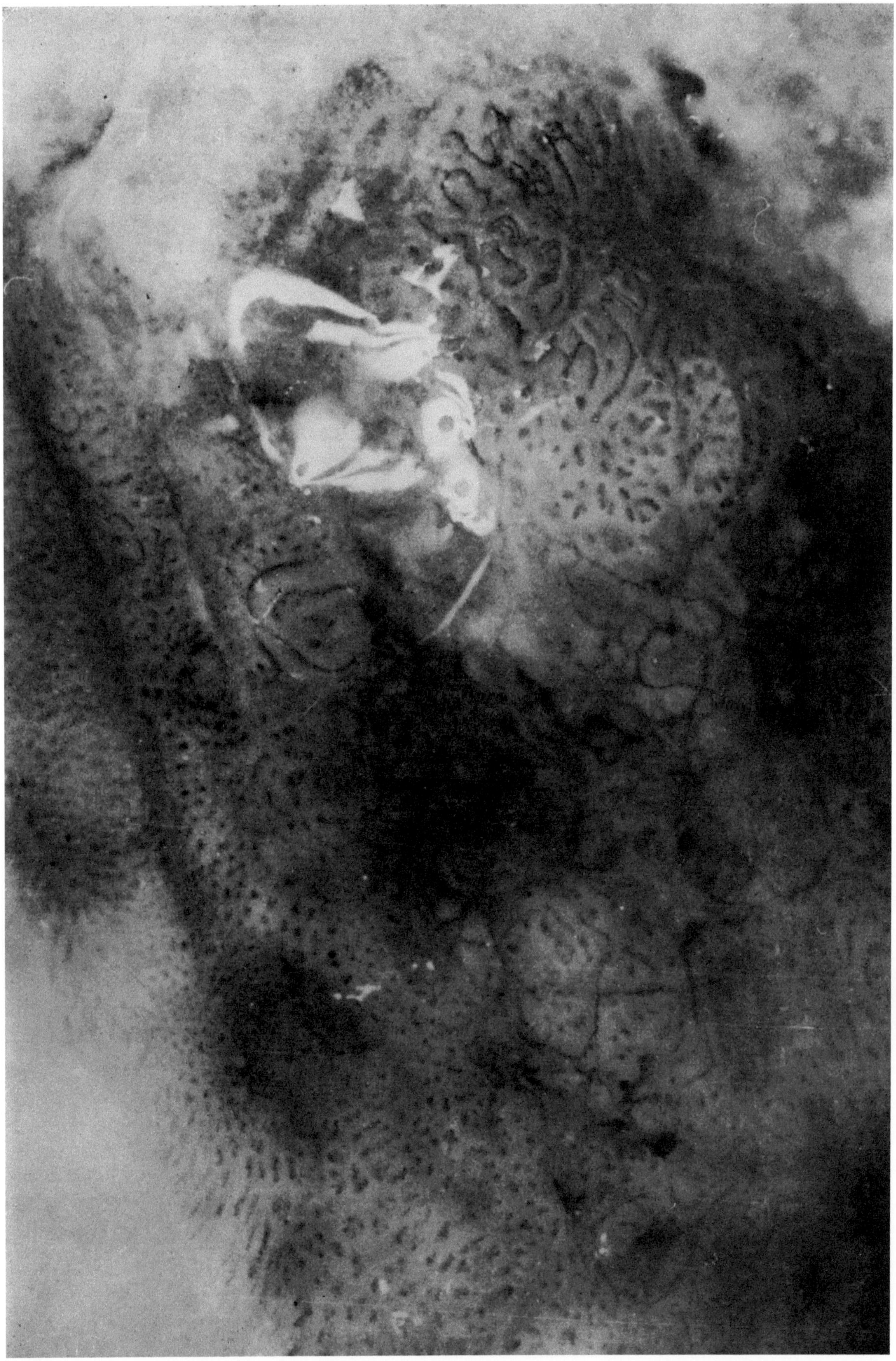

Plate 22 Punctuation, mosaic, atypical vessels

Atypical hairpin vessels, corresponding to simple and papillary floor, and atypical network capillaries of bizarre field pattern as well as larger intercapillary spacings, vascular irregularity, and difference in levels seem to suggest presence of early invasive carcinoma.

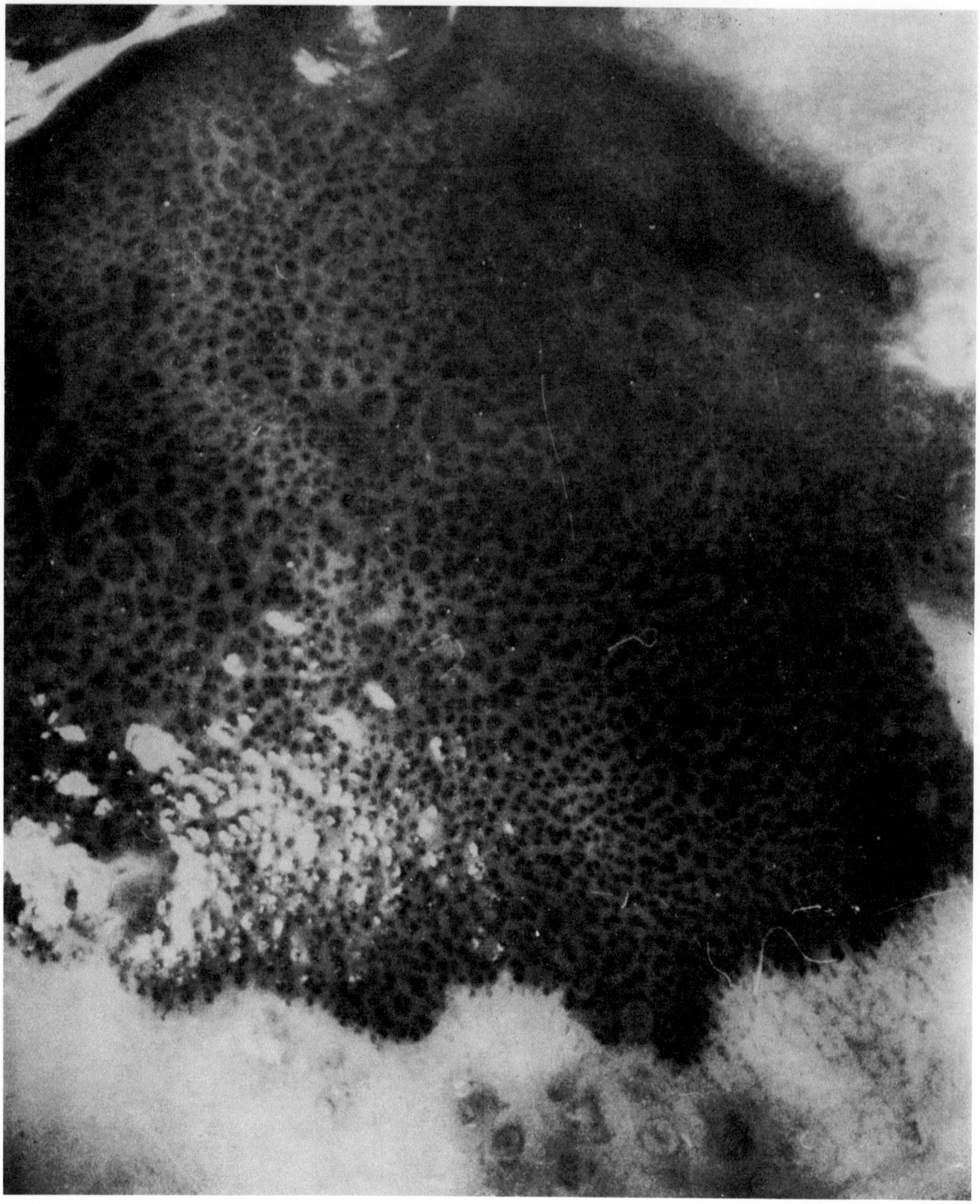

Plate 23 **Punctuation, atypical vessels, and invasive carcinoma**

Vessels originating from atypical hairpin capillaries of papillary floor in proliferating bed of invasive carcinoma; some vessels arranged to exhibit "carcinomatous negative field pattern".

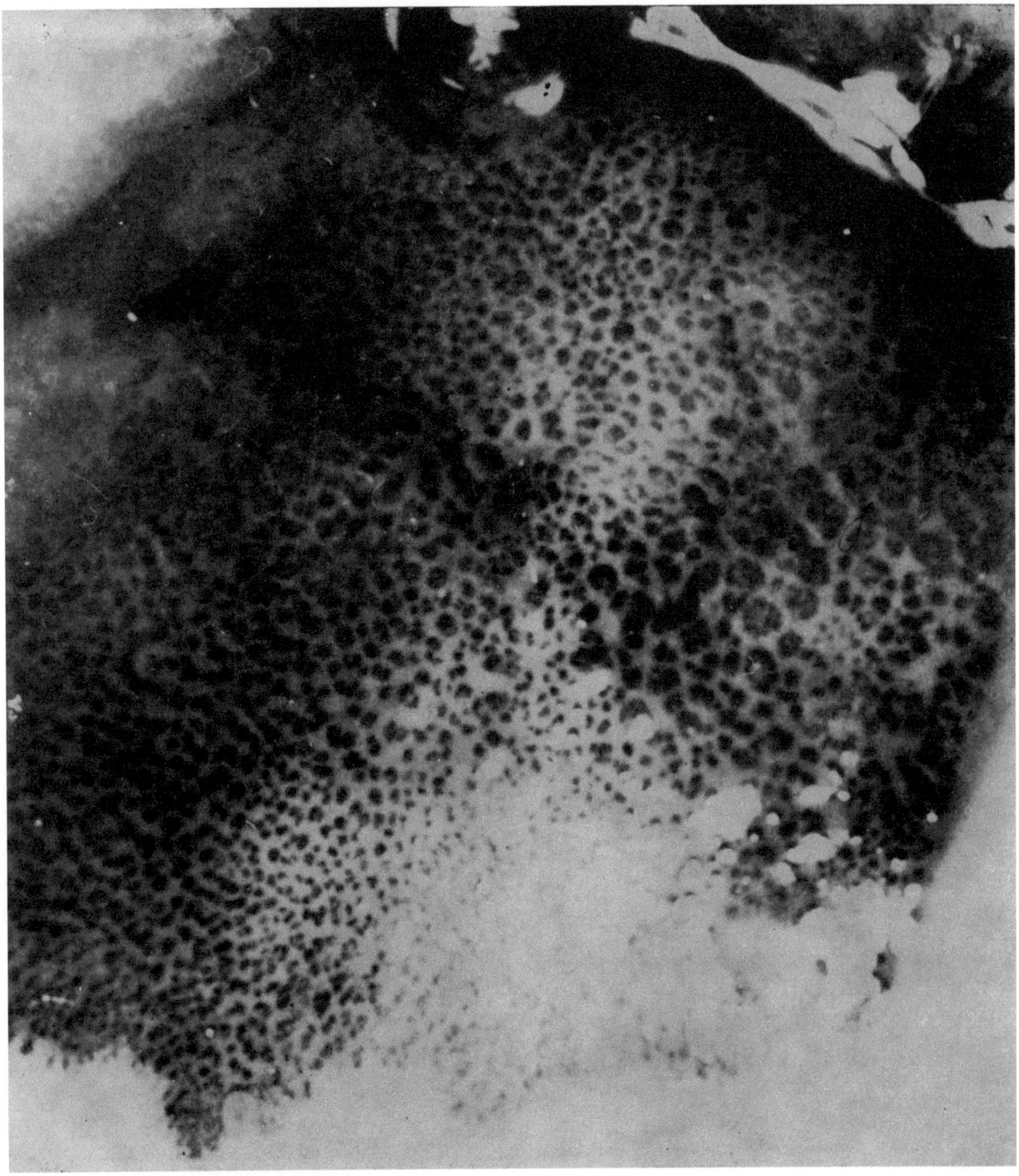

Plate 24 **Punctuation, atypical, vessels, carcinoma**
Stepwise ascension of vascular irregularity, depending on transformation of tissue.

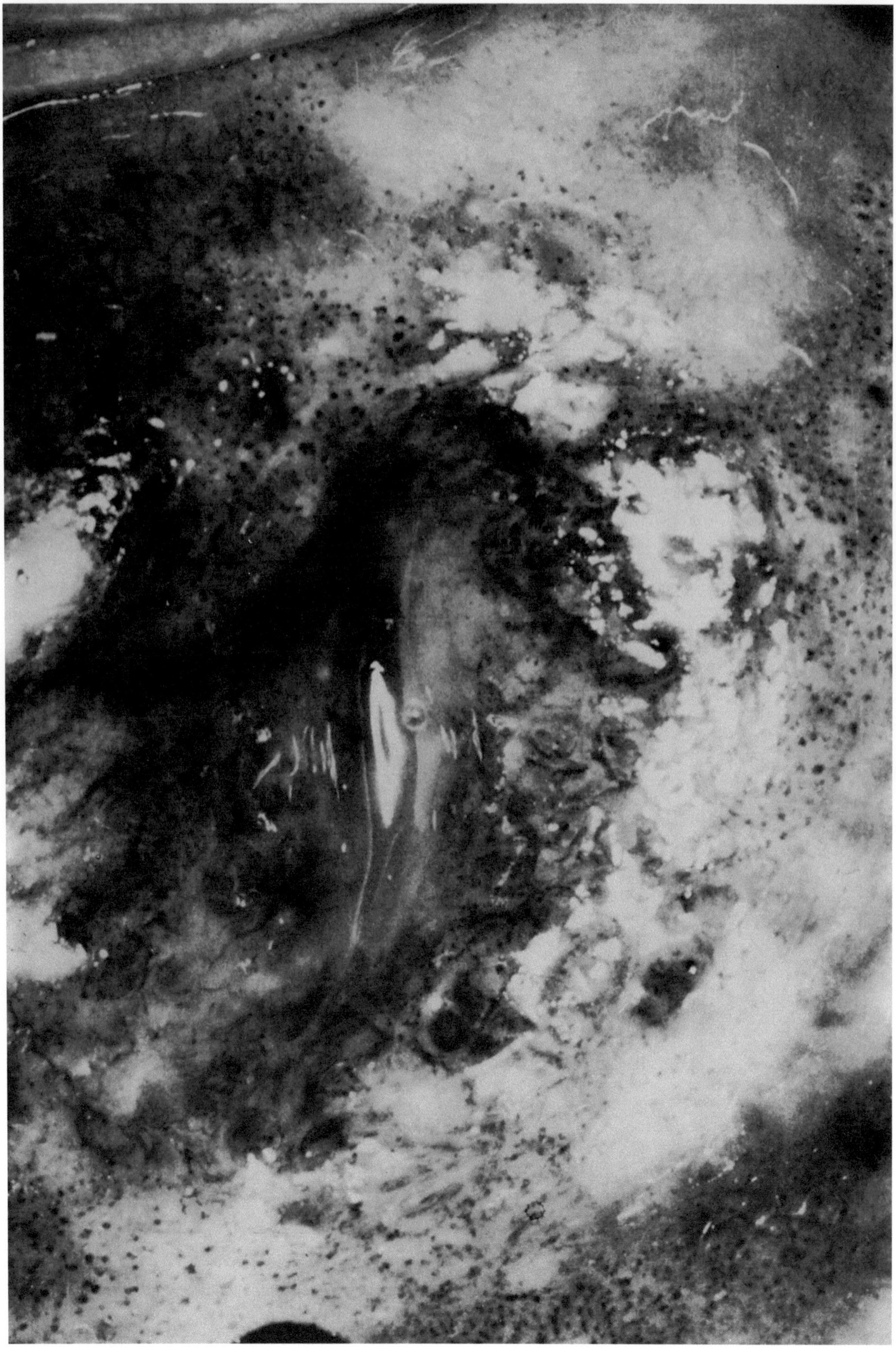

Plate 25 **Punctuation, carcinoma**
Simple and papillary floor regions as marginal areas of carcinogenesis in CZ; indicator function of what is called matrix regions!

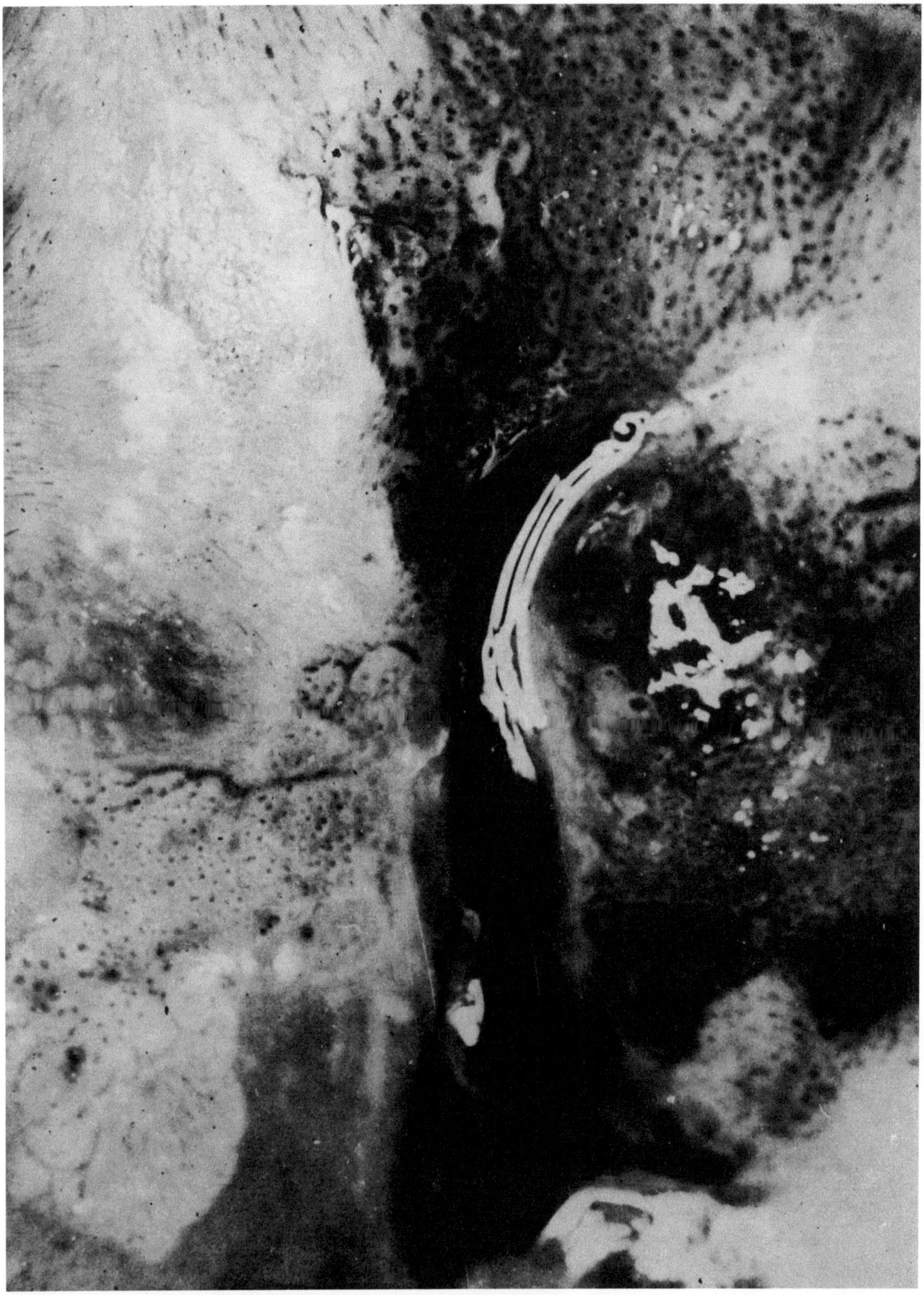

Plate 26 Punctuation, mosaic, atypical vessels, and white epithelium
Remarkable parallelism of simple and papillary floor, field pattern regions, vinegar-white metaplastic epithelium, and open, keratinised, warped glandular outlets.

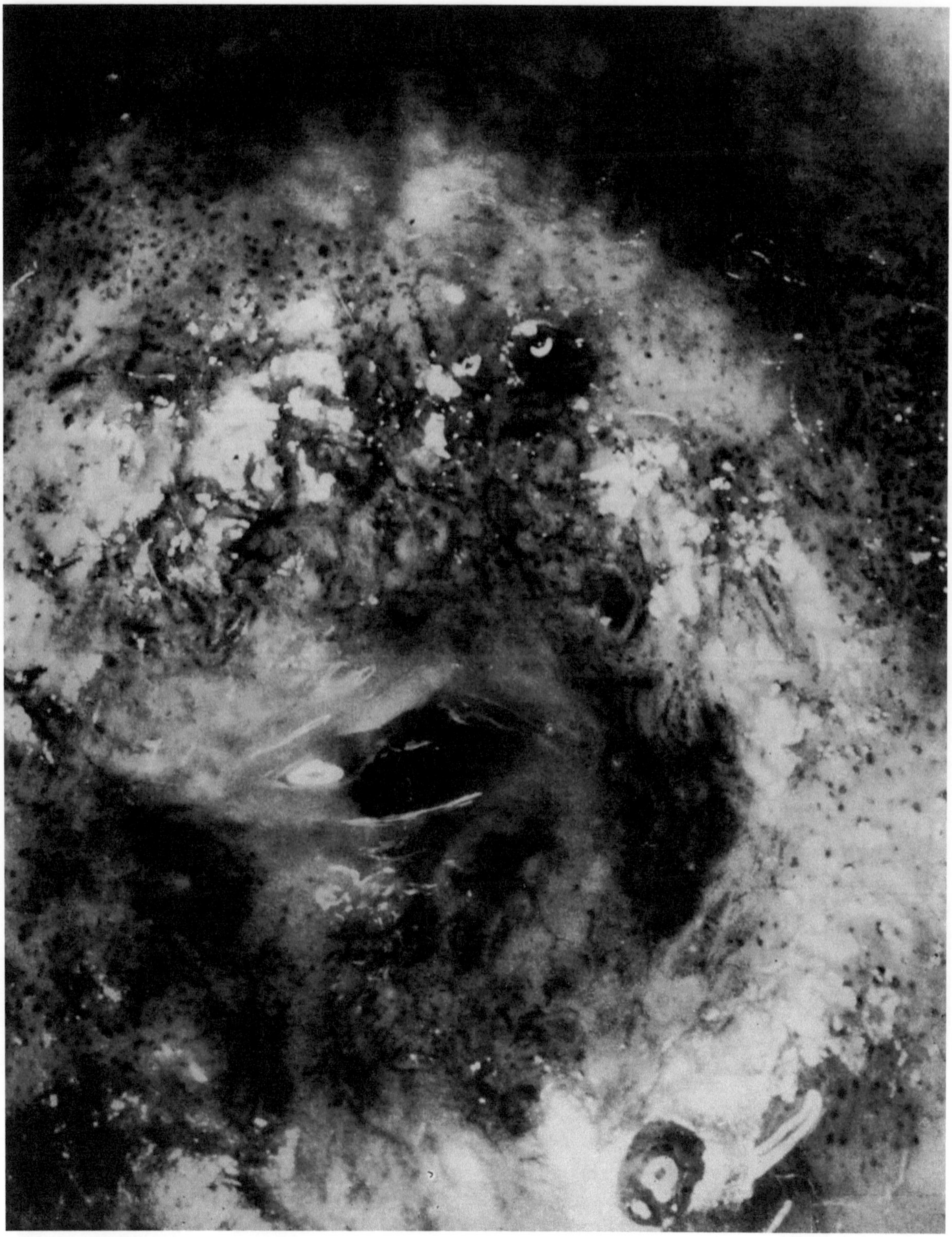

Plate 27 **Atypical vessels, keratosis, and carcinoma**
Carcinoma vessels originating from vessels of floor and field pattern structures; conspicuously washed-out appearance of carcinoma.

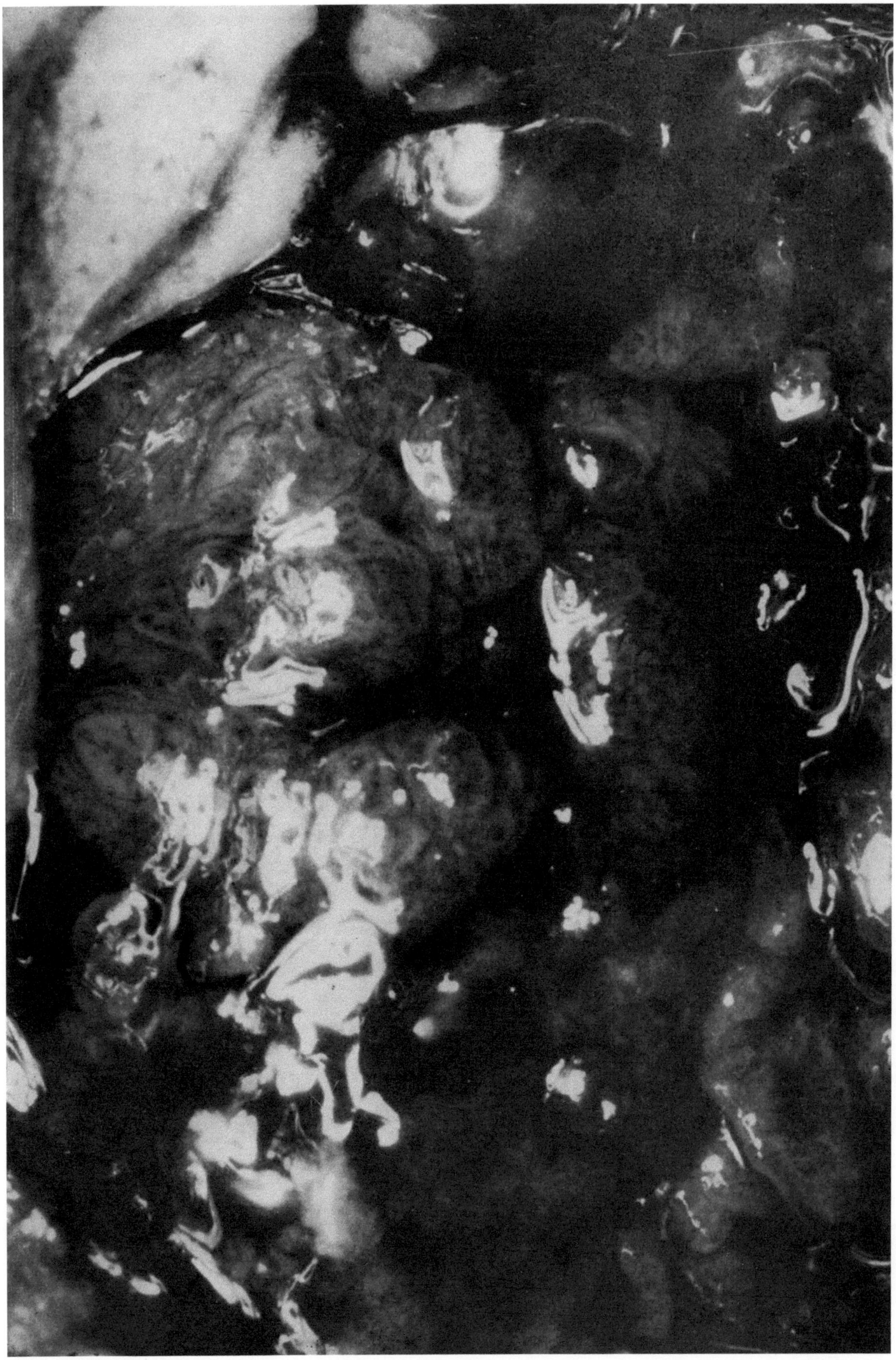

Plate 28 **Keratosis, atypical vessels, carcinoma**
Exophytically growing carcinoma, giving superficial impression of polypus

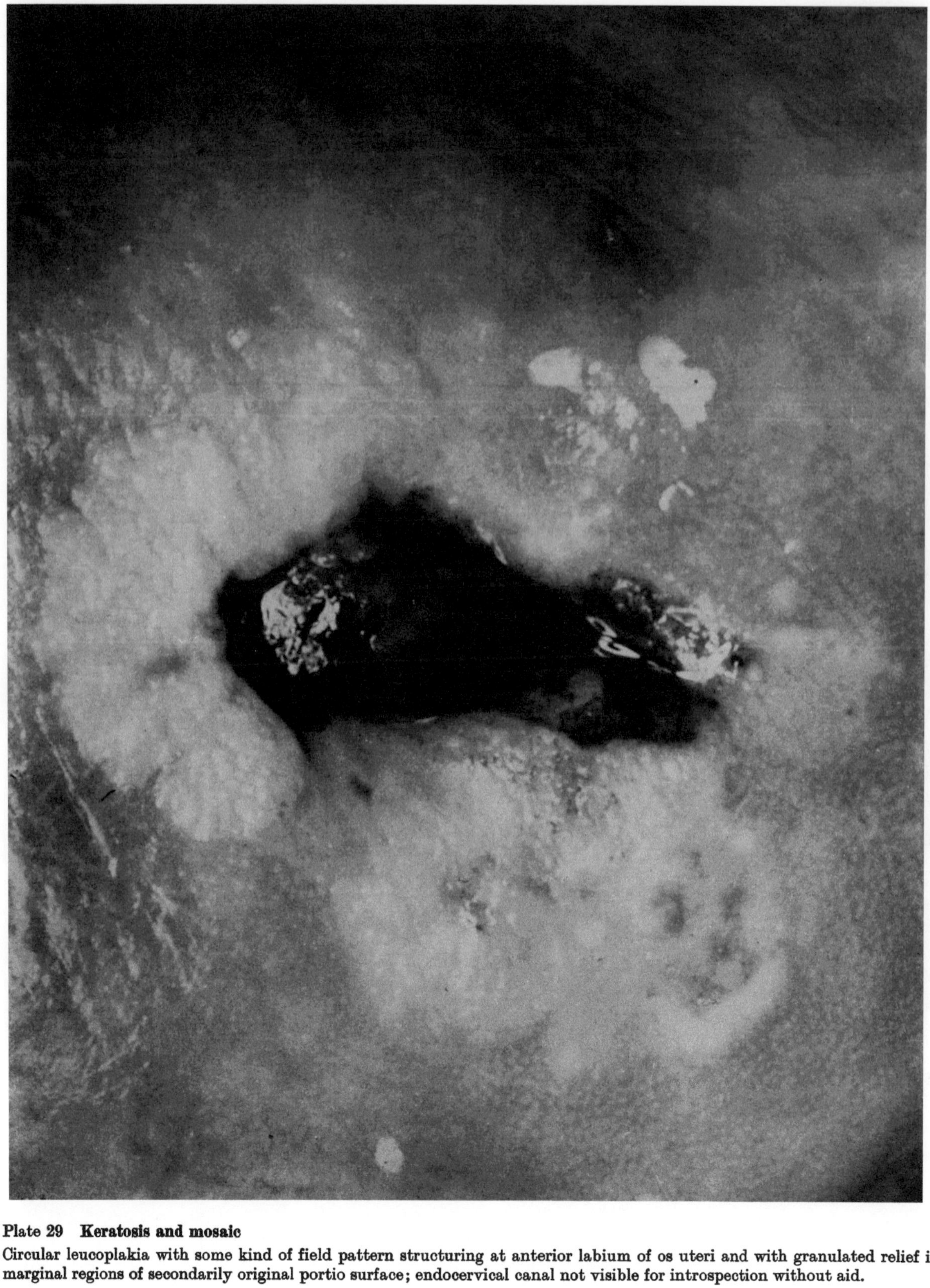

Plate 29 Keratosis and mosaic

Circular leucoplakia with some kind of field pattern structuring at anterior labium of os uteri and with granulated relief in marginal regions of secondarily original portio surface; endocervical canal not visible for introspection without aid.

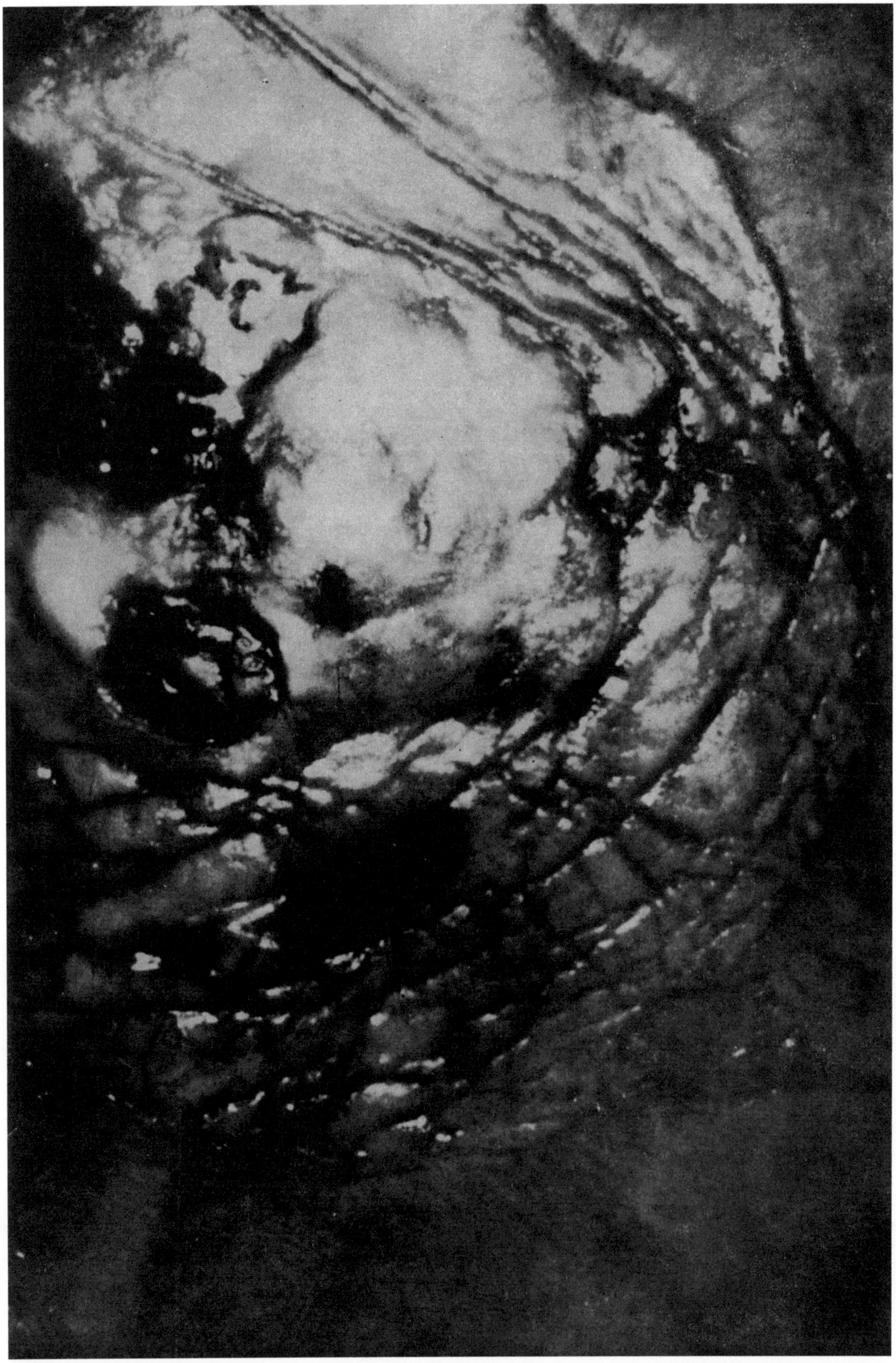

Plate 30 **Keratosis and mosaic**
Excessive keratinisation changing, in marginal regions, to squamous leucoplakia and, finally, to keratinising field pattern; epithelial defect, surface topography, and expansion suggest presence of somewhat severe atypia.

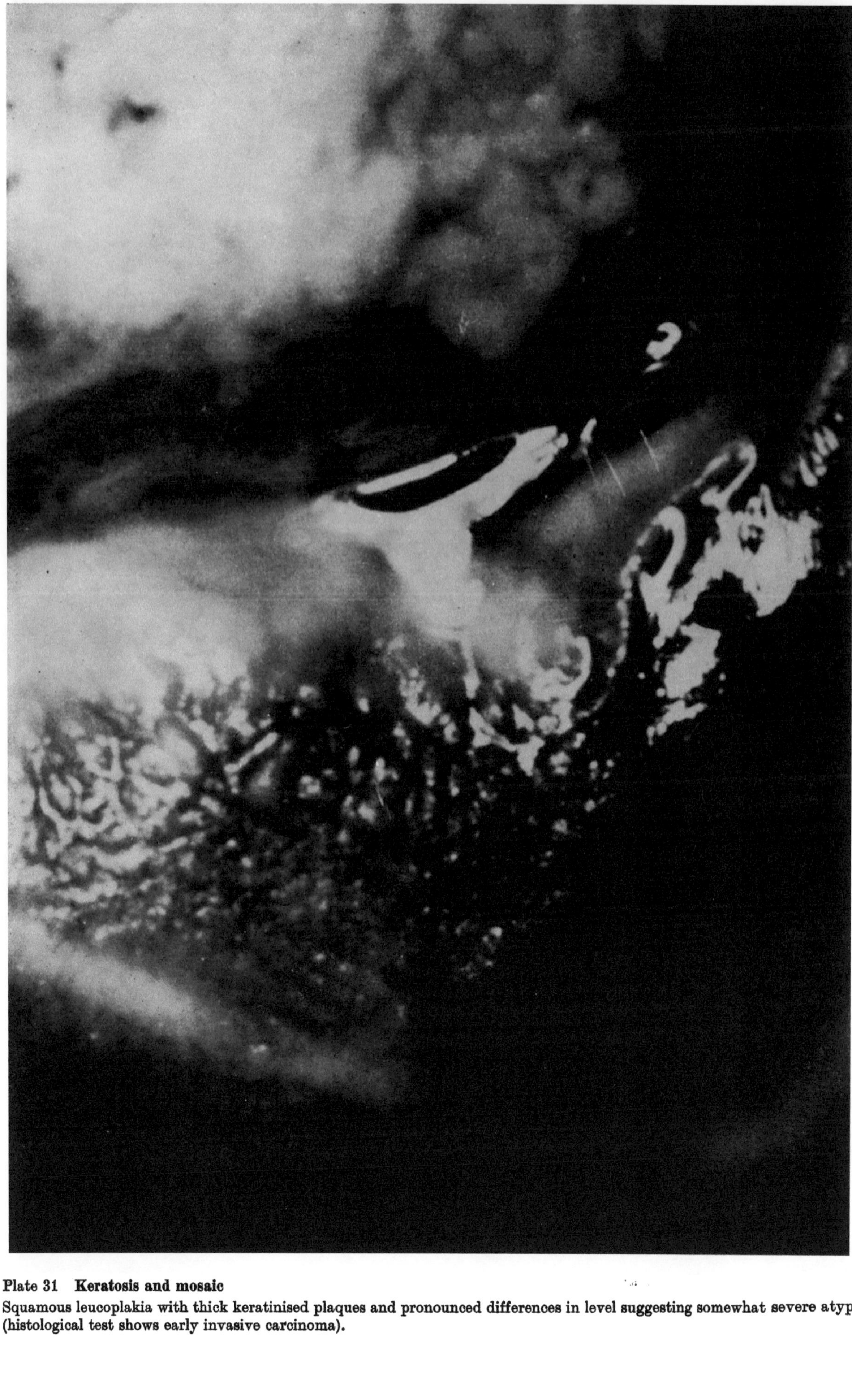

Plate 31 Keratosis and mosaic
Squamous leucoplakia with thick keratinised plaques and pronounced differences in level suggesting somewhat severe atypia (histological test shows early invasive carcinoma).

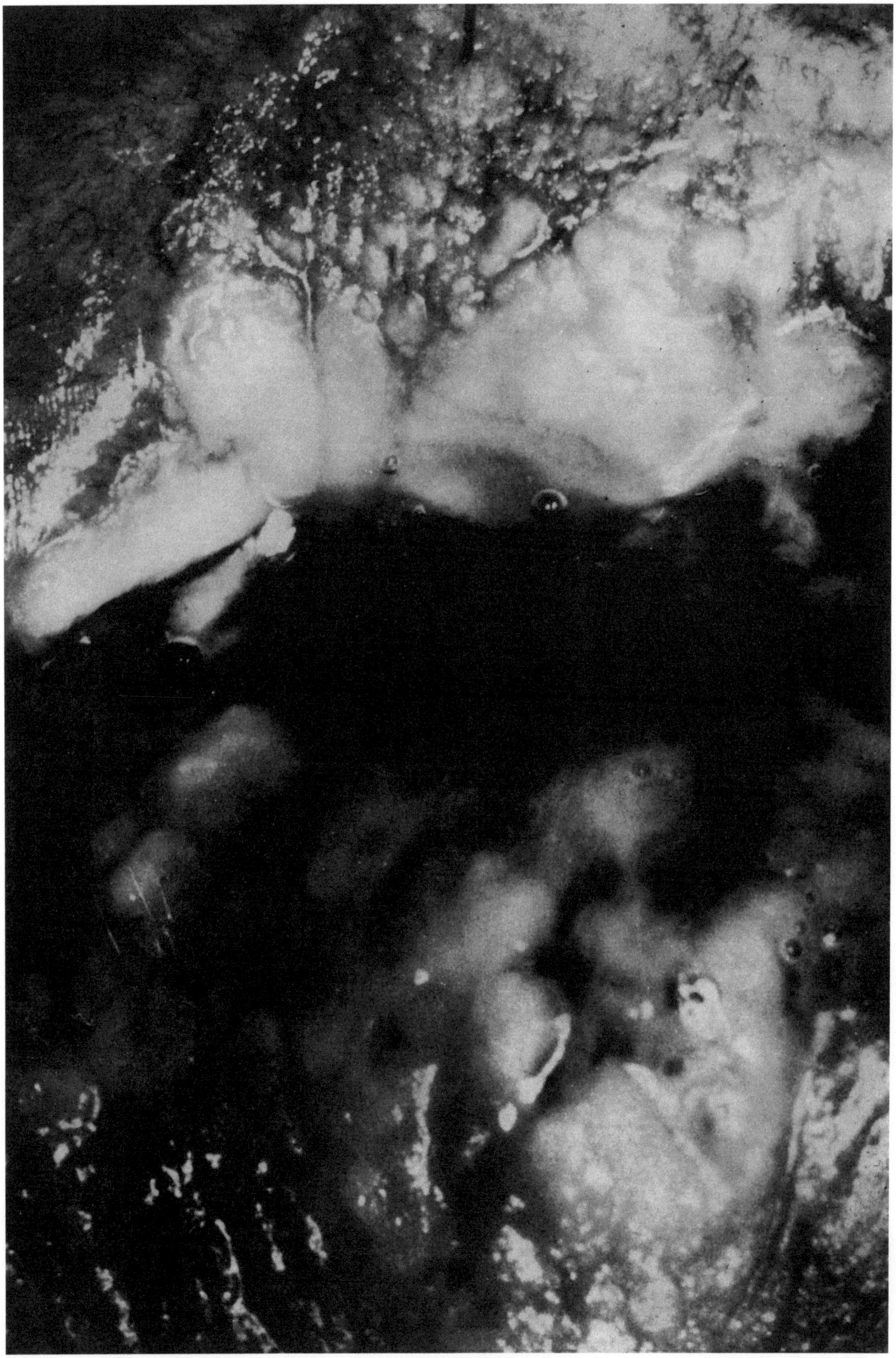

Plate 32 Keratosis and mosaic

Leucoplakia with extreme plaque formation and slightly indicated keratinised field pattern; vascular diagnosis possible only in marginal regions (histological test shows early invasive carcinoma).

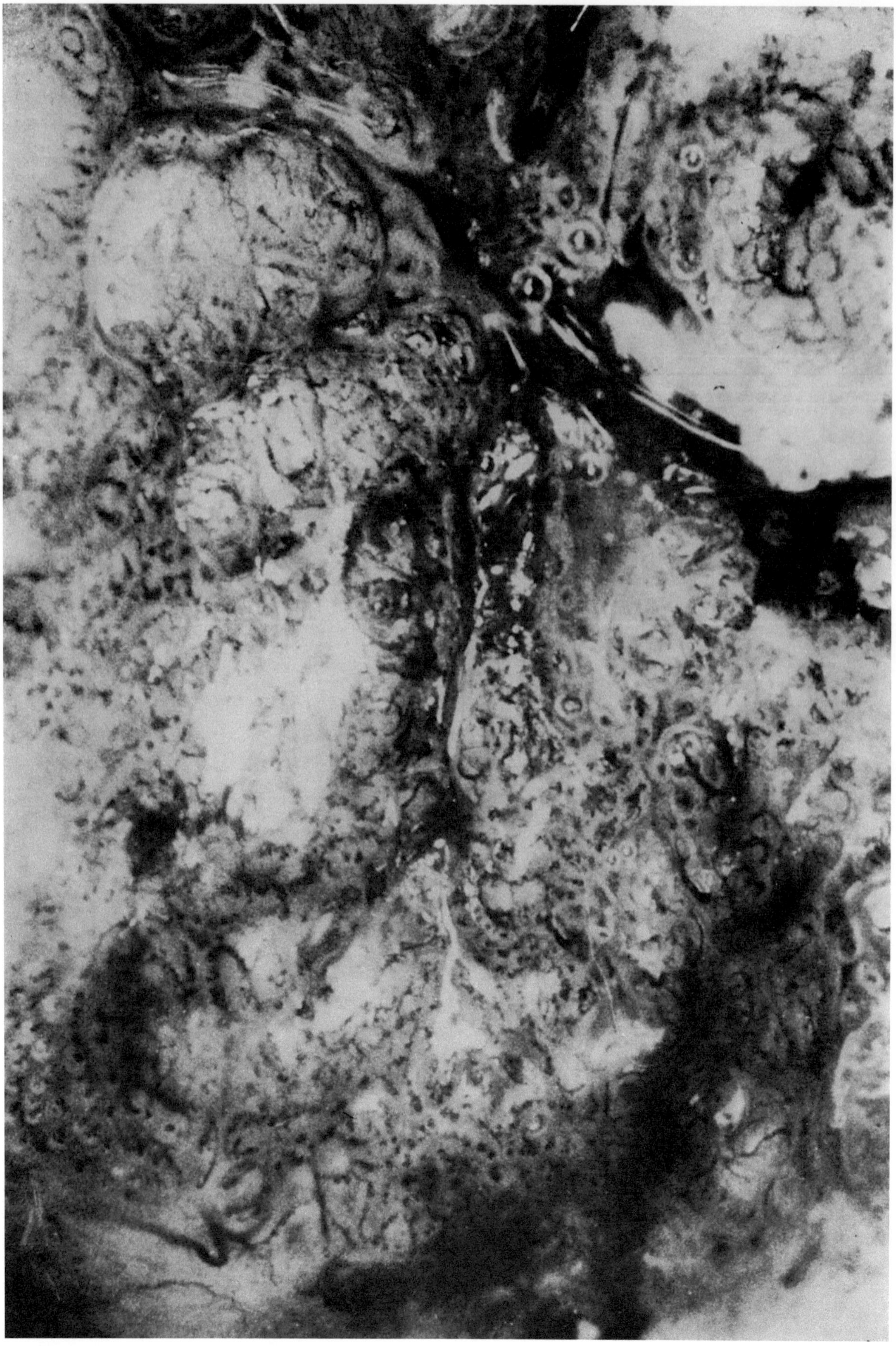

Plate 33 Mosaic, punctuation, and atypical vessels

Field pattern and papillary floor regions as well as atypical hairpin capillaries, loops, and comma-shaped vessels, all with pronounced difference in level; presence of early invasive carcinoma suggested by intercapillary spacings, according to *Koller* and *Kolstad* (histologically confirmed).

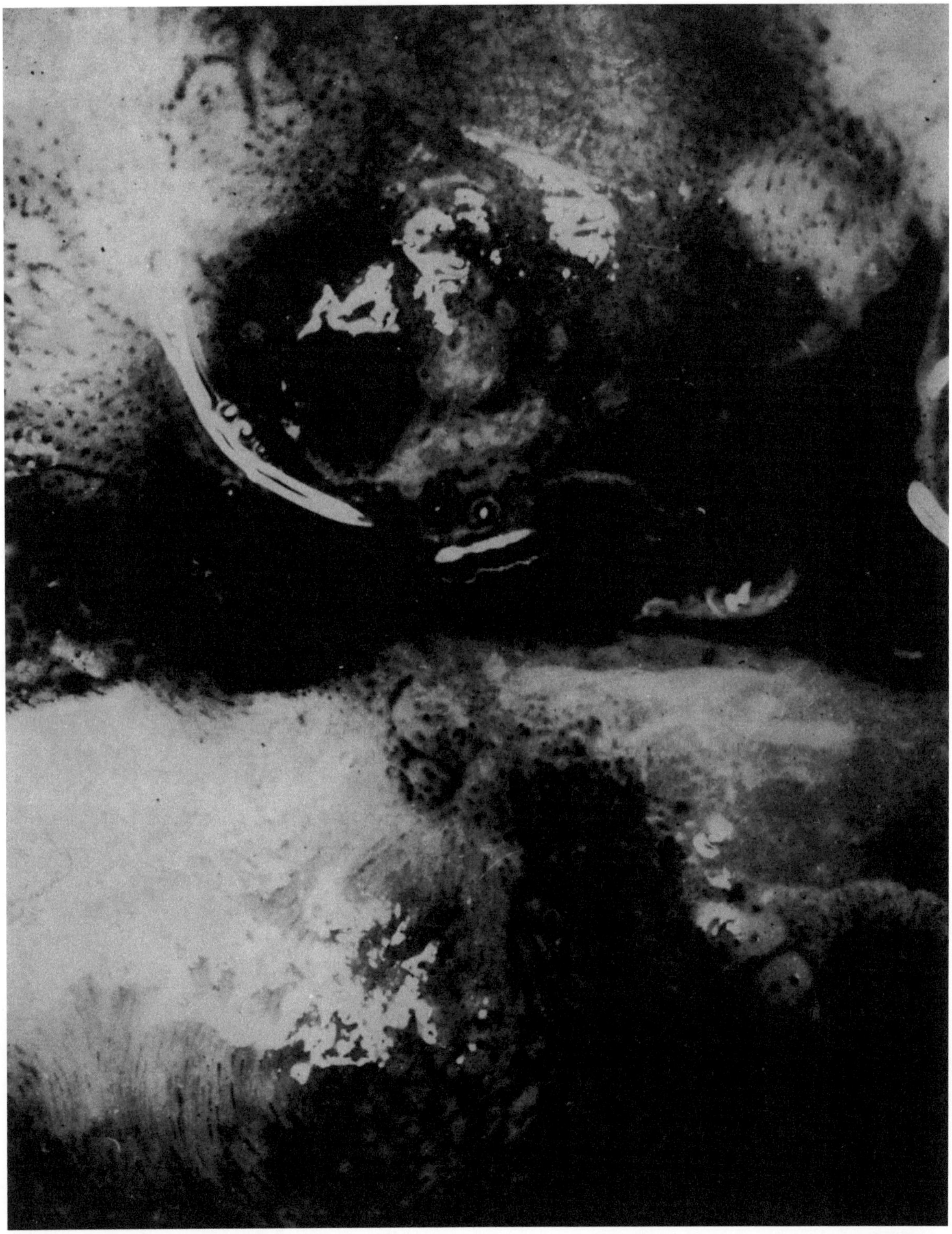

Plate 34 Punctuation and mosaic

Atypsical hairpin capillaries at posterior labium of os uteri, giving impression of simple and papillary floor; histologically established carcinoma in situ; papillary floor areas and raised field pattern at anterior labium of os uteri; histologically established early invasion of stroma

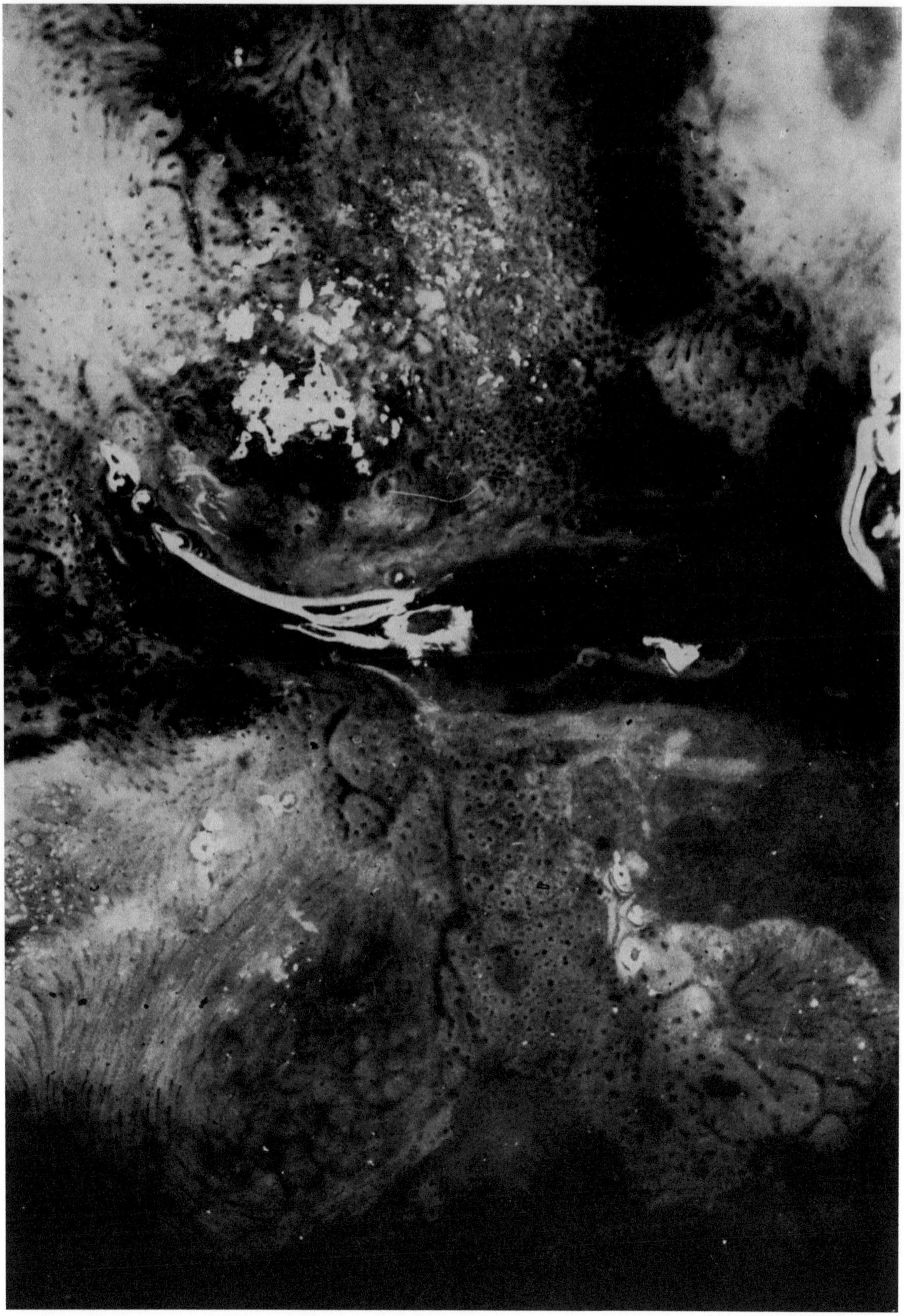

Plate 35 Punctuation, mosaic, and white epithelium

Rare complexity of parallel existence of simple and papillary floor, simple, raised, and keratinised field pattern, as well as incipient exophytism; conspicuously aggravated trend to haemorrhage; differences between epithelial levels.

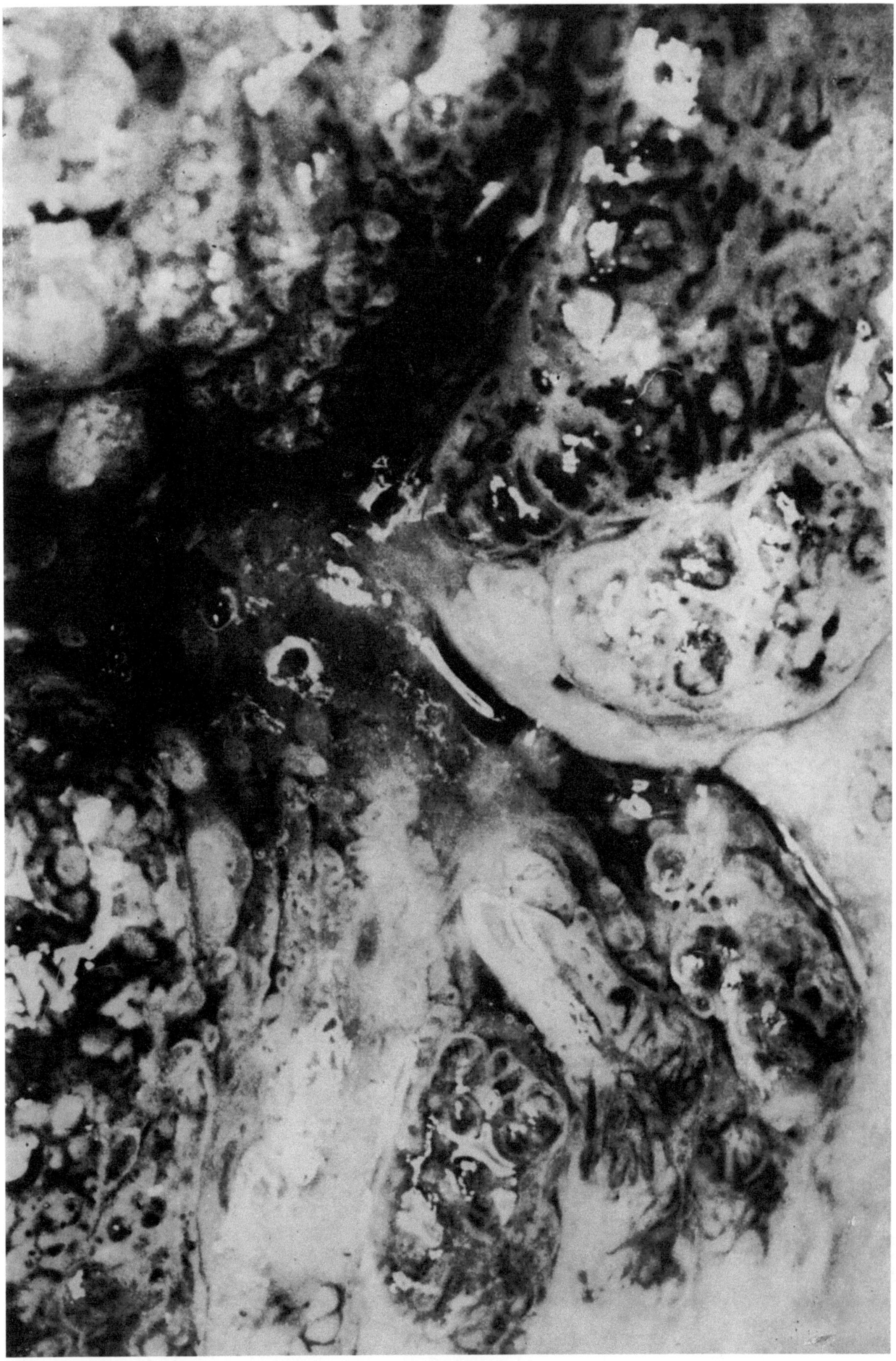

Plate 36 Mosaic, punctuation, atypical vessels, and carcinoma

Atypical vessels differ from ectopic vessels by usually being clearly visible, following use of acetic acid which, therefore, should be used, whenever diagnosis has to be backed up.

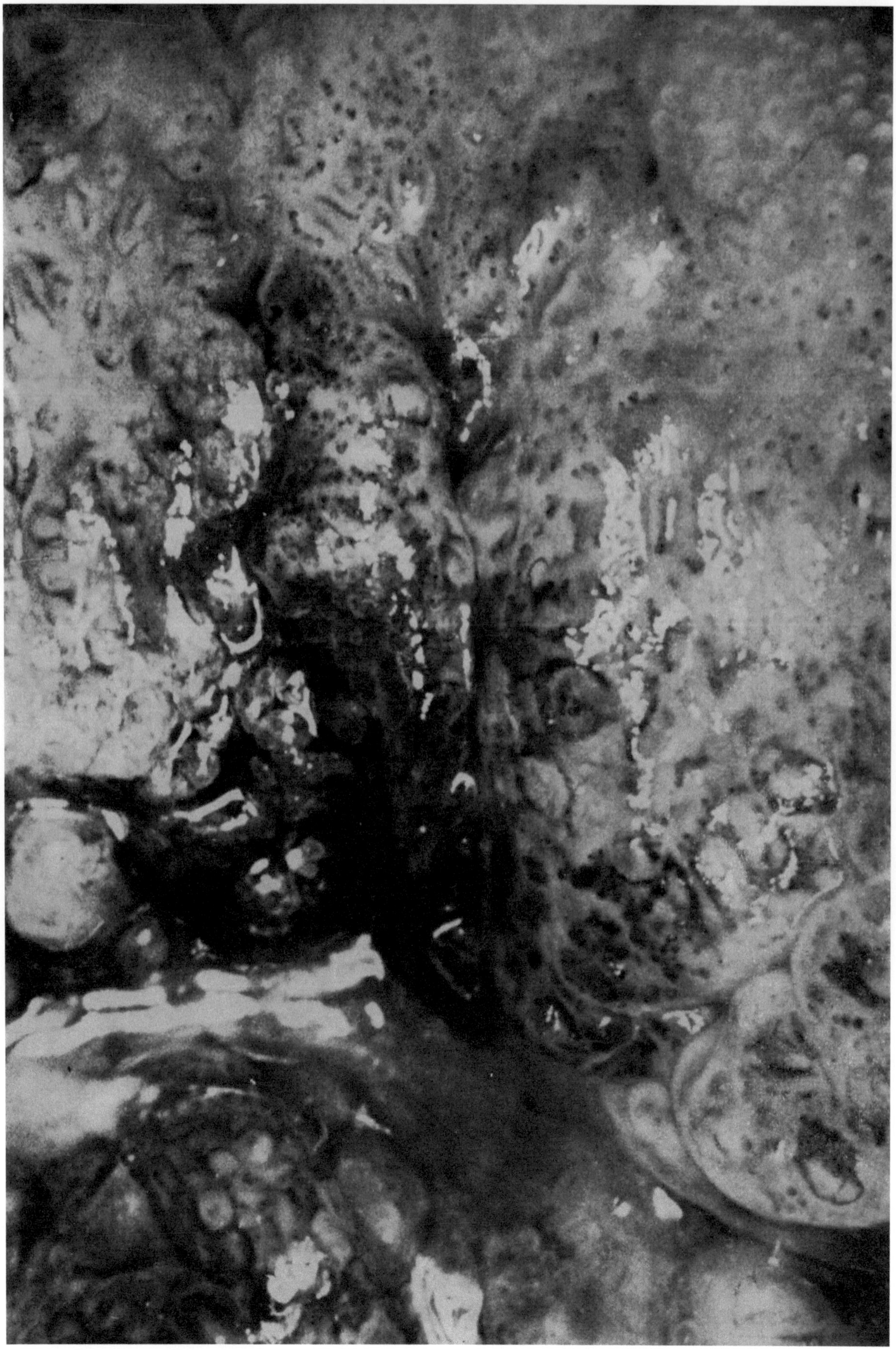

Plate 37 **Mosaic and punctuation**
Clear fading of epithelium causing clear pronunciation of atypical vessels.

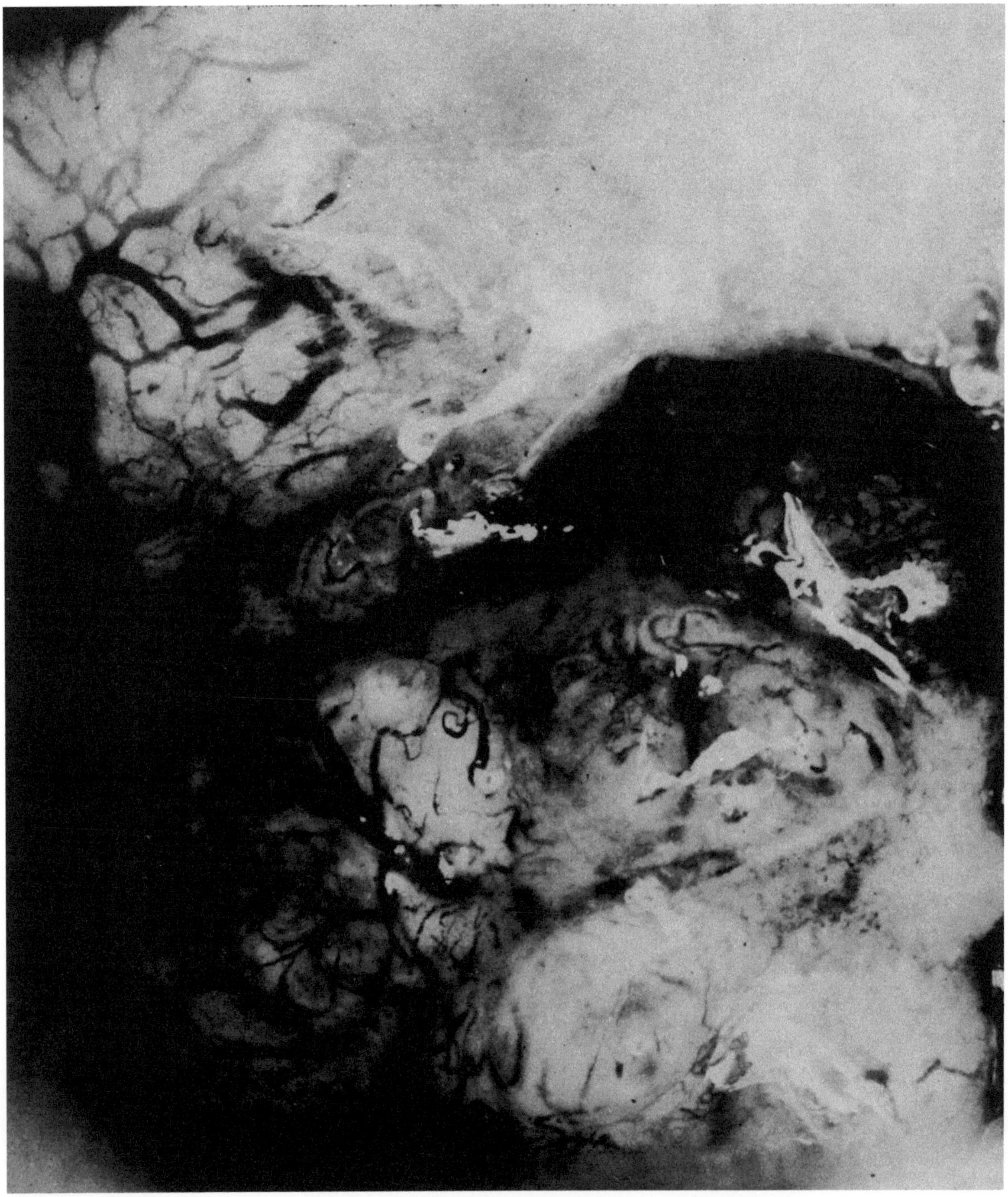

Plate 38 Atypical vessels and invasive carcinoma

Most important criteria of original invasive carcinoma visible in minute detail: variation and disruption of calibres, angiectasia, bizarre vessel lines, avascular areas, atypical vascular arborisation, and formation of anastomoses.

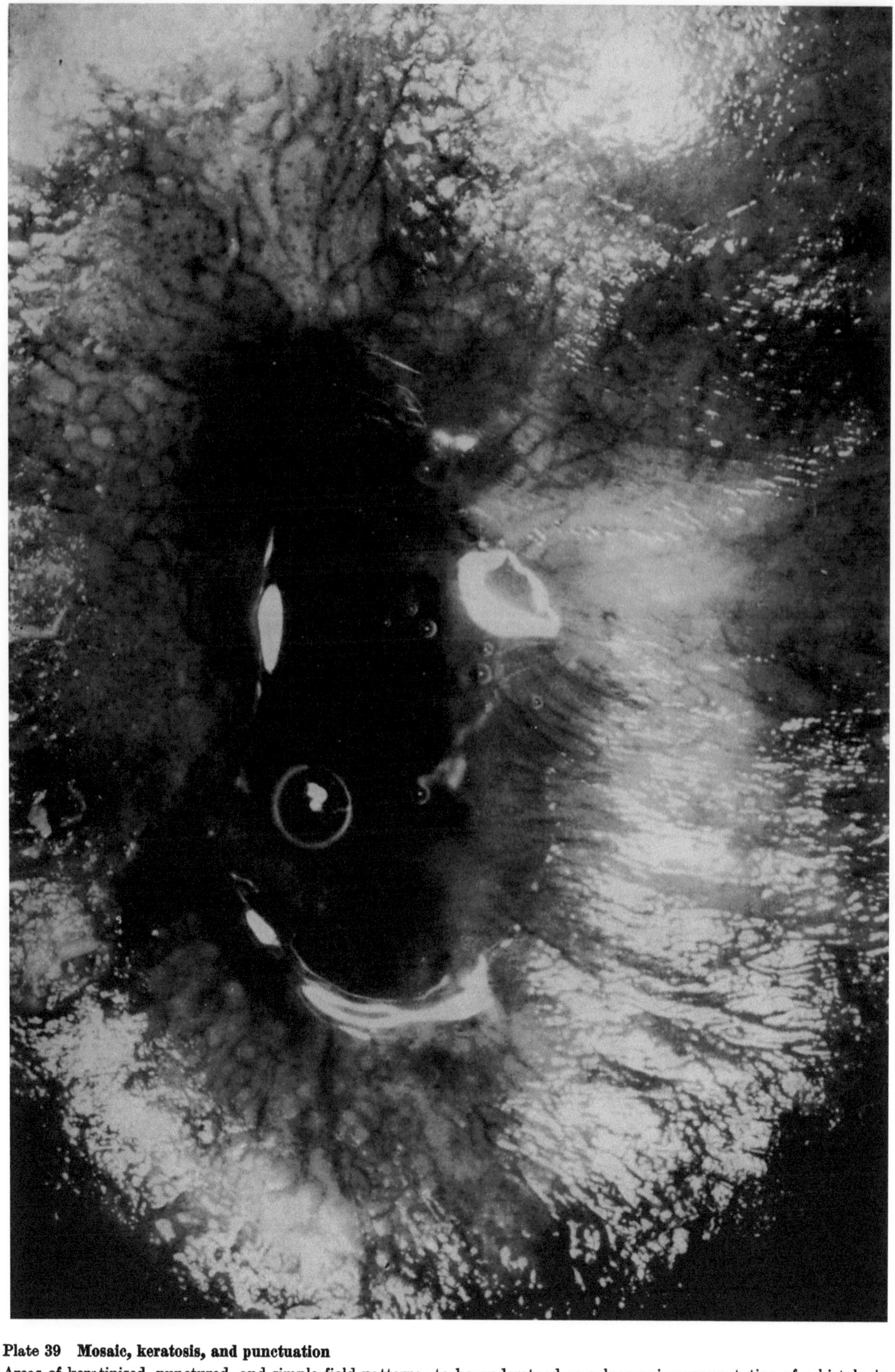

Plate 39 Mosaic, keratosis, and punctuation

Areas of keratinised, punctured, and simple field patterns; to be understood as colposcopic representation of a histological picture in which atypical epithelium is found to be located in connective tissue or in "glands" beneath level of surface epithelium; field patterns shown as whitish-opaque tissue areas separated from each other by red vascular connective tissue septa with thin epithelium on top of them.

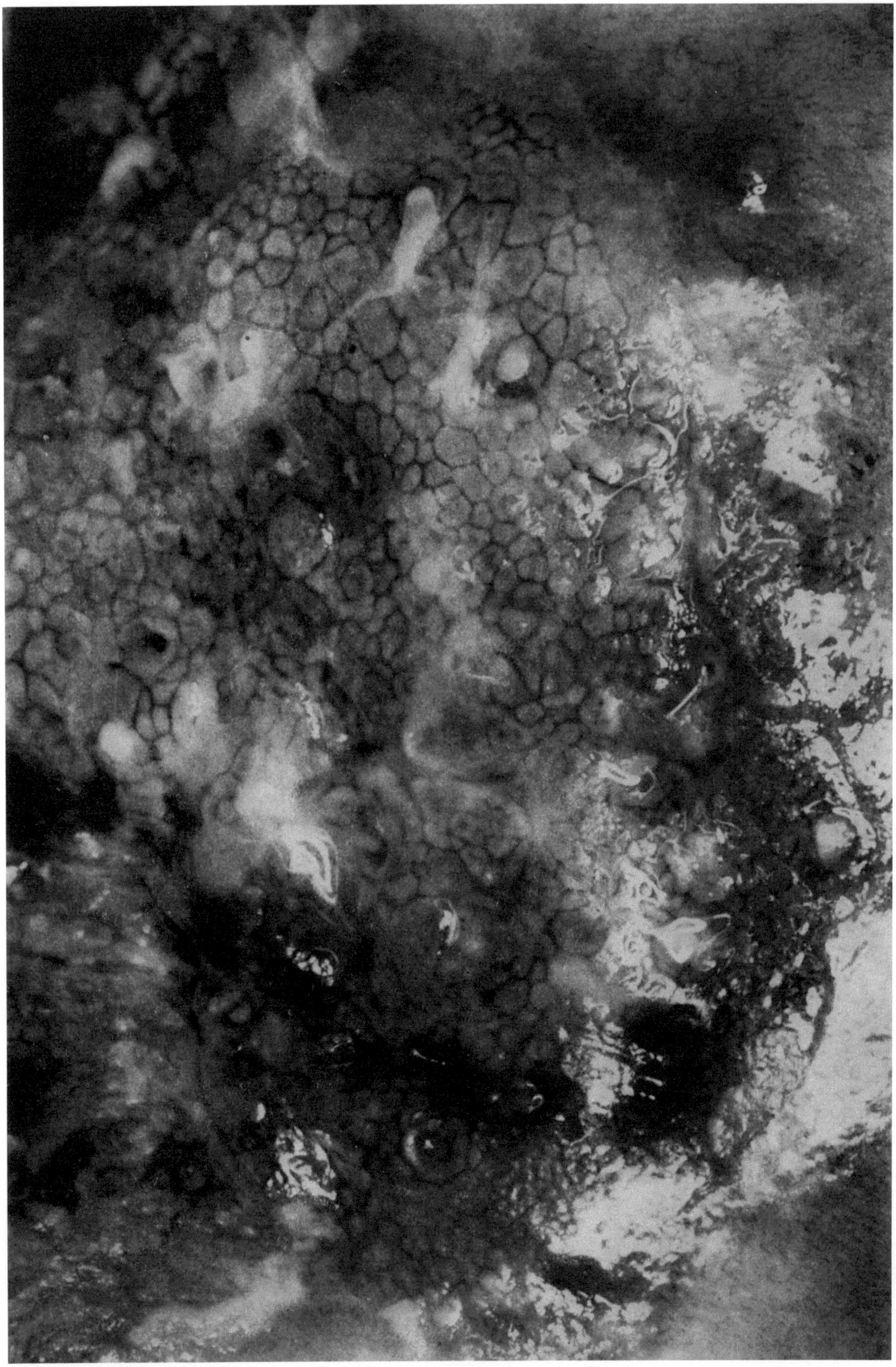

Plate 40 **Mosaic, keratosis**

Polygonal field patterns changing in size and shape; drastic difference, by 100 per cent, between intercapillary spacings; some fields keratinised, similar to "funnel field pattern", described in this Atlas; other fields show open glandular outlets.

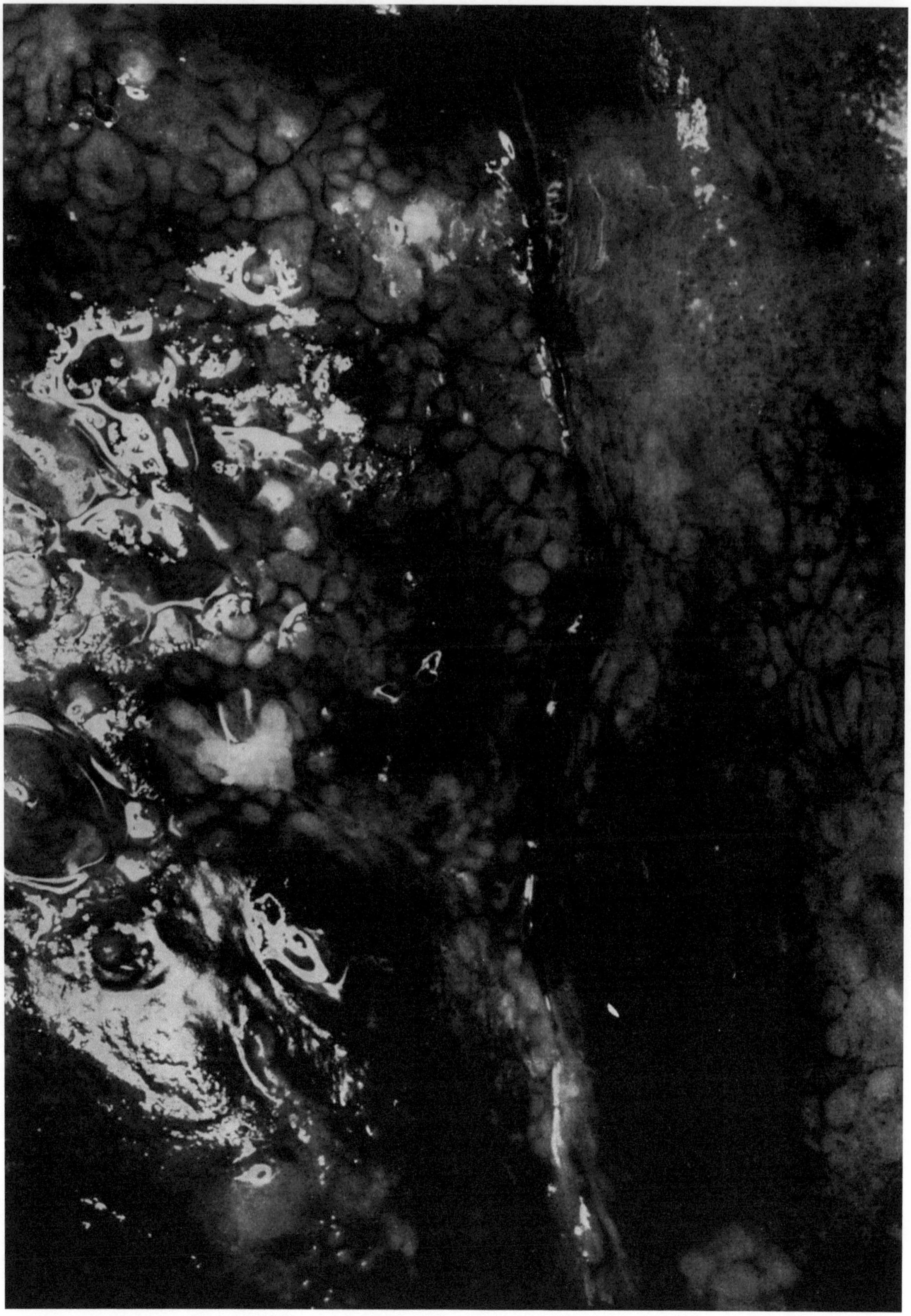

Plate 41 **Mosaic, keratosis, punctuation, atypical vessels, carcinoma**

Irregular field pattern structures with trend to keratinisation; open keratinised glandular outlets; excessive trend to haemorrhage; differences in level according to exophytic and endophytic processes; papillary floor regions in right upper part of Plate; colposcopic diagnosis of invasive carcinoma histologically confirmed.

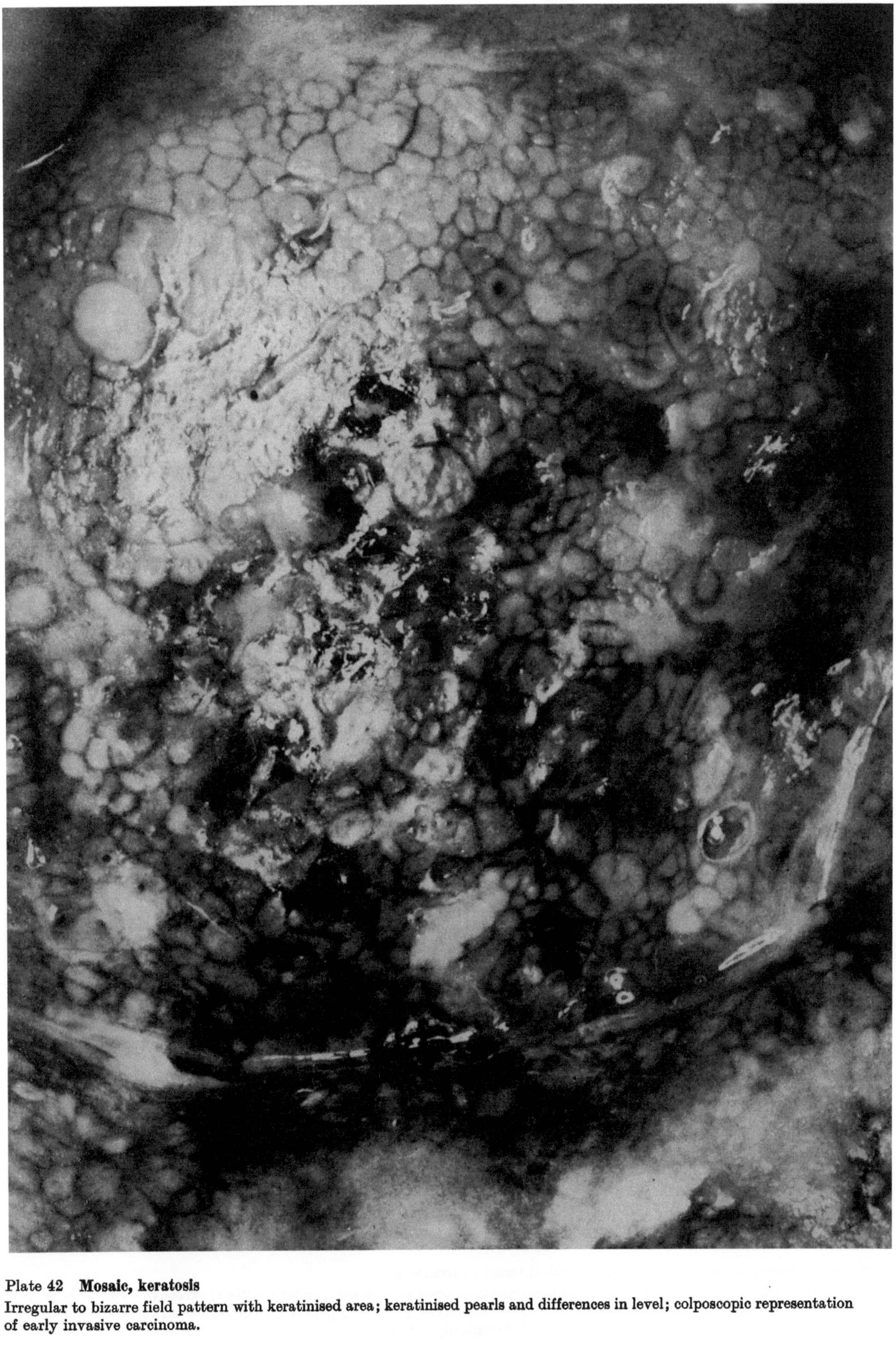

Plate 42 **Mosaic, keratosis**
Irregular to bizarre field pattern with keratinised area; keratinised pearls and differences in level; colposcopic representation of early invasive carcinoma.

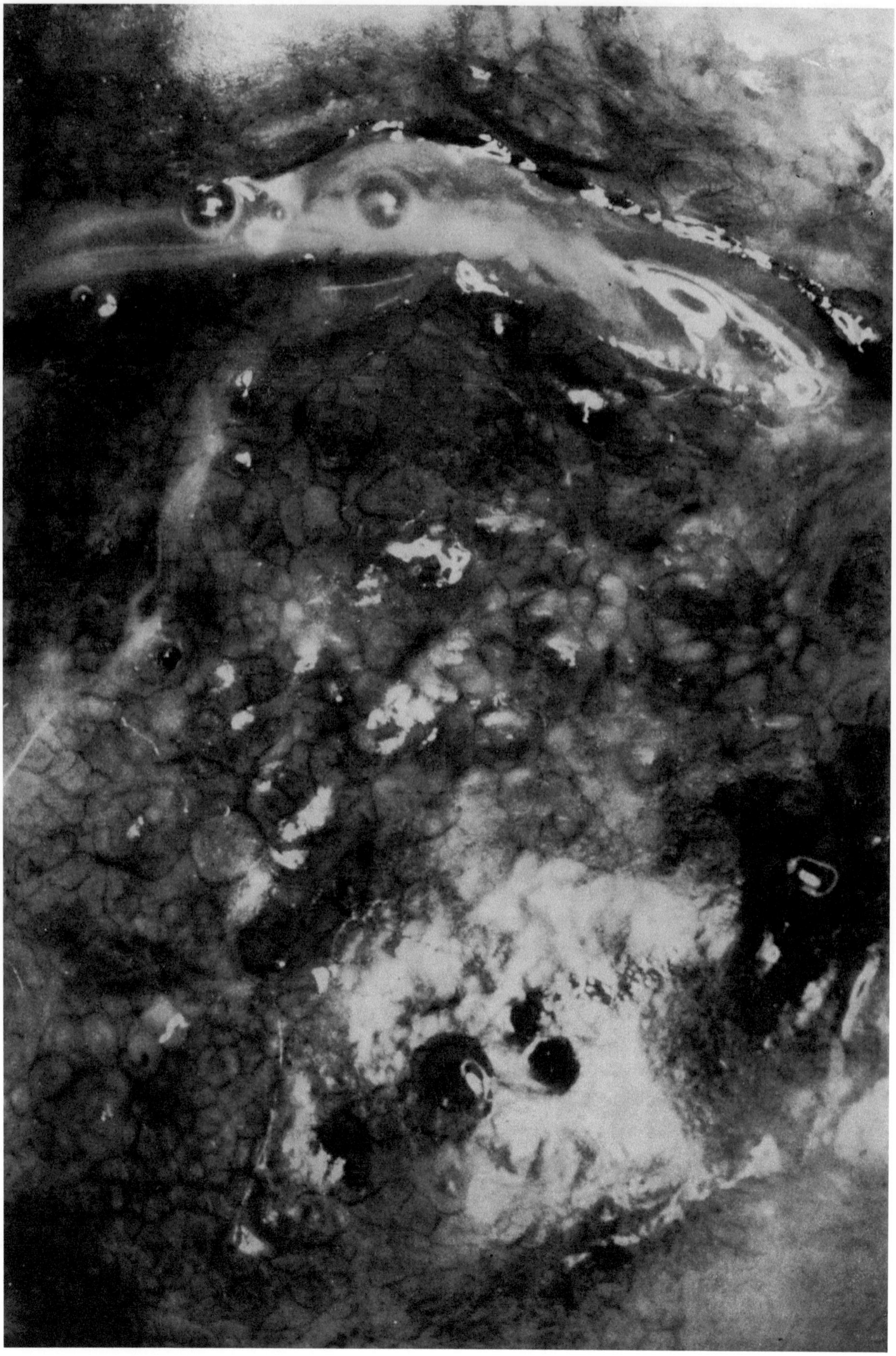

Plate 43 Mosaic, keratosis

Irregular, bizarre field pattern with relatively large mosaic fields changing in shape, with glands entrapped in some of them; atypical nature of histological findings aggravating along with atypical vessels in connective tissue septa of fields.

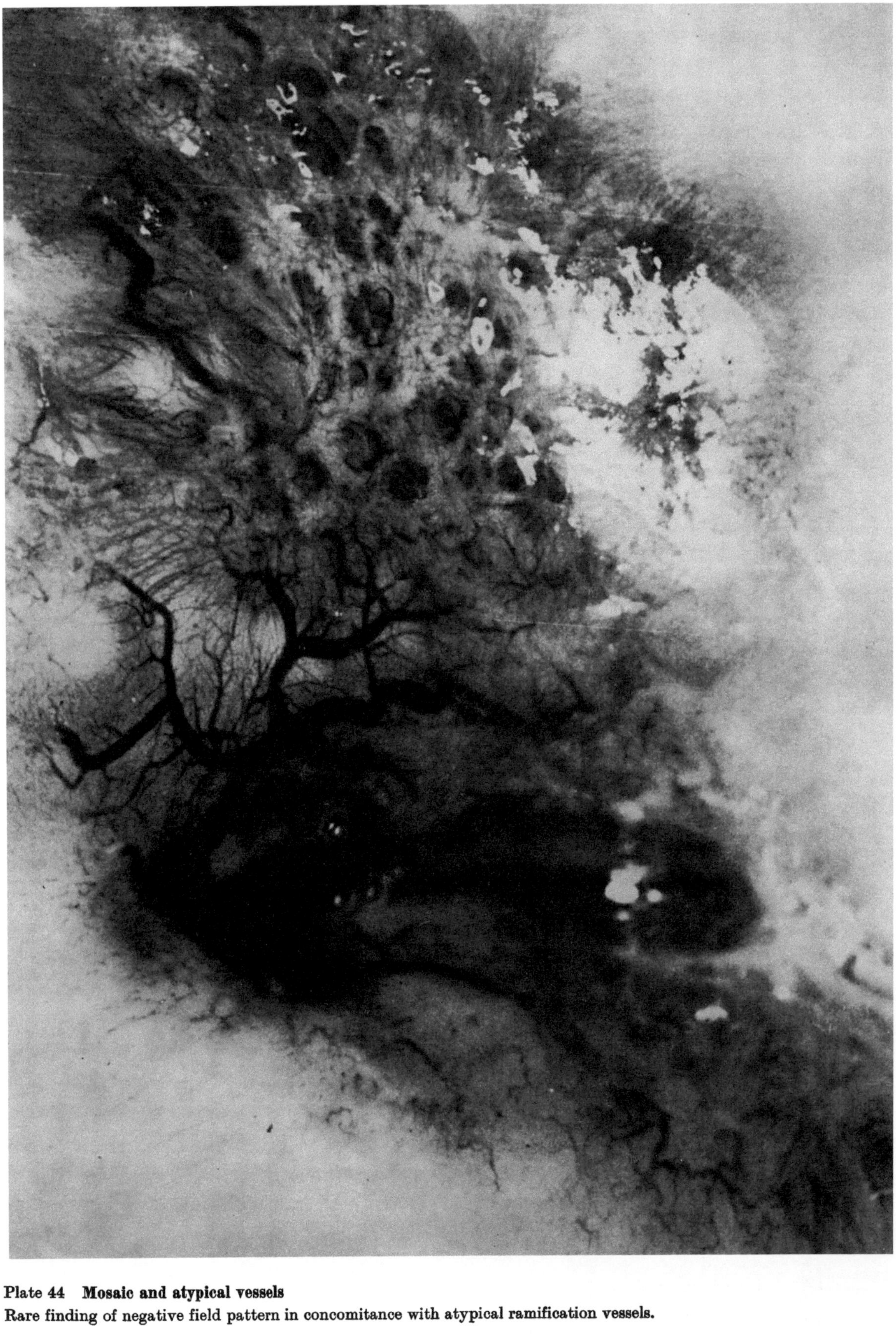

Plate 44 Mosaic and atypical vessels
Rare finding of negative field pattern in concomitance with atypical ramification vessels.

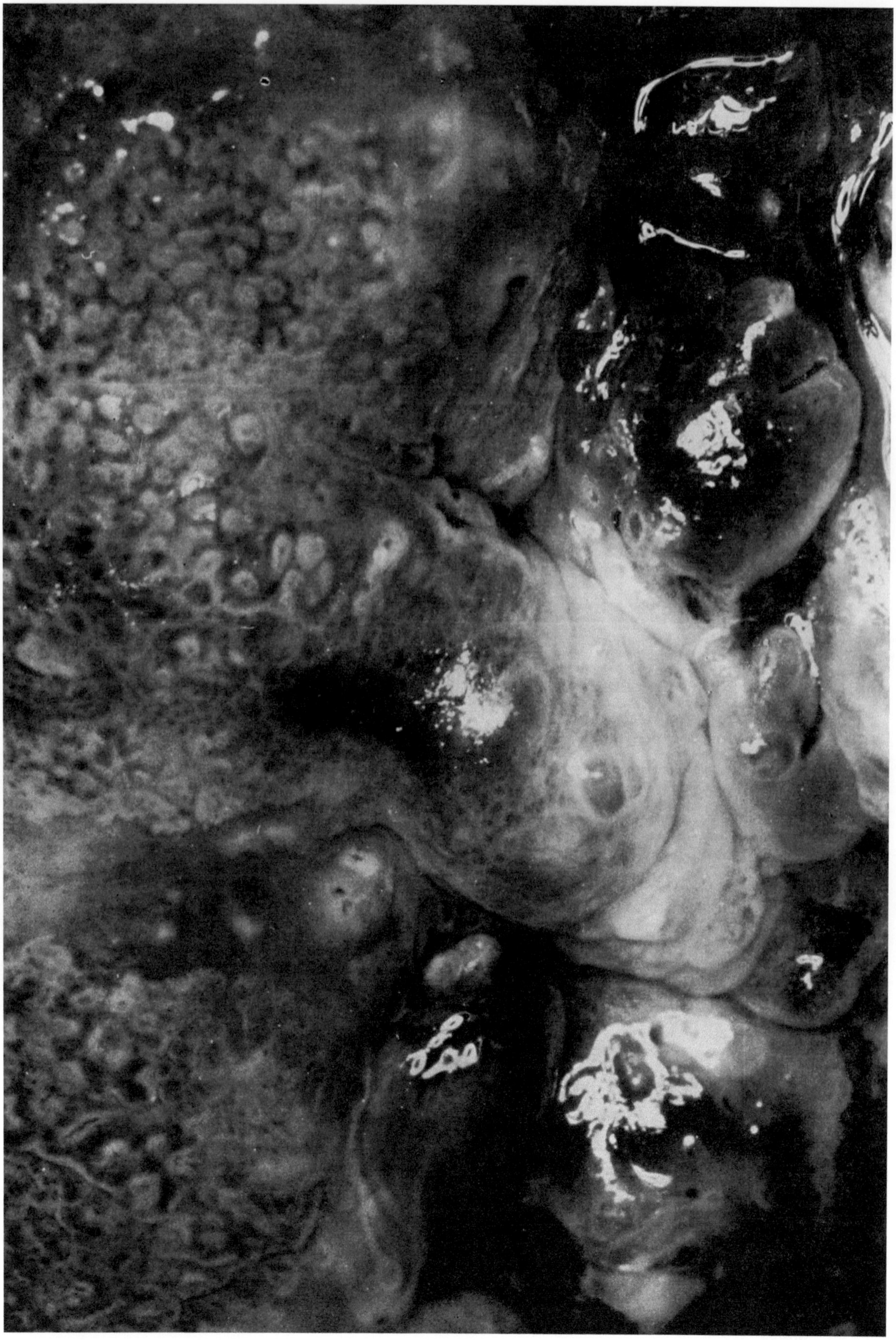

Plate 45 Mosaic and carcinoma
Clearly pronounced areas with raised and negative field patterns in marginal regions of invasive carcinoma.

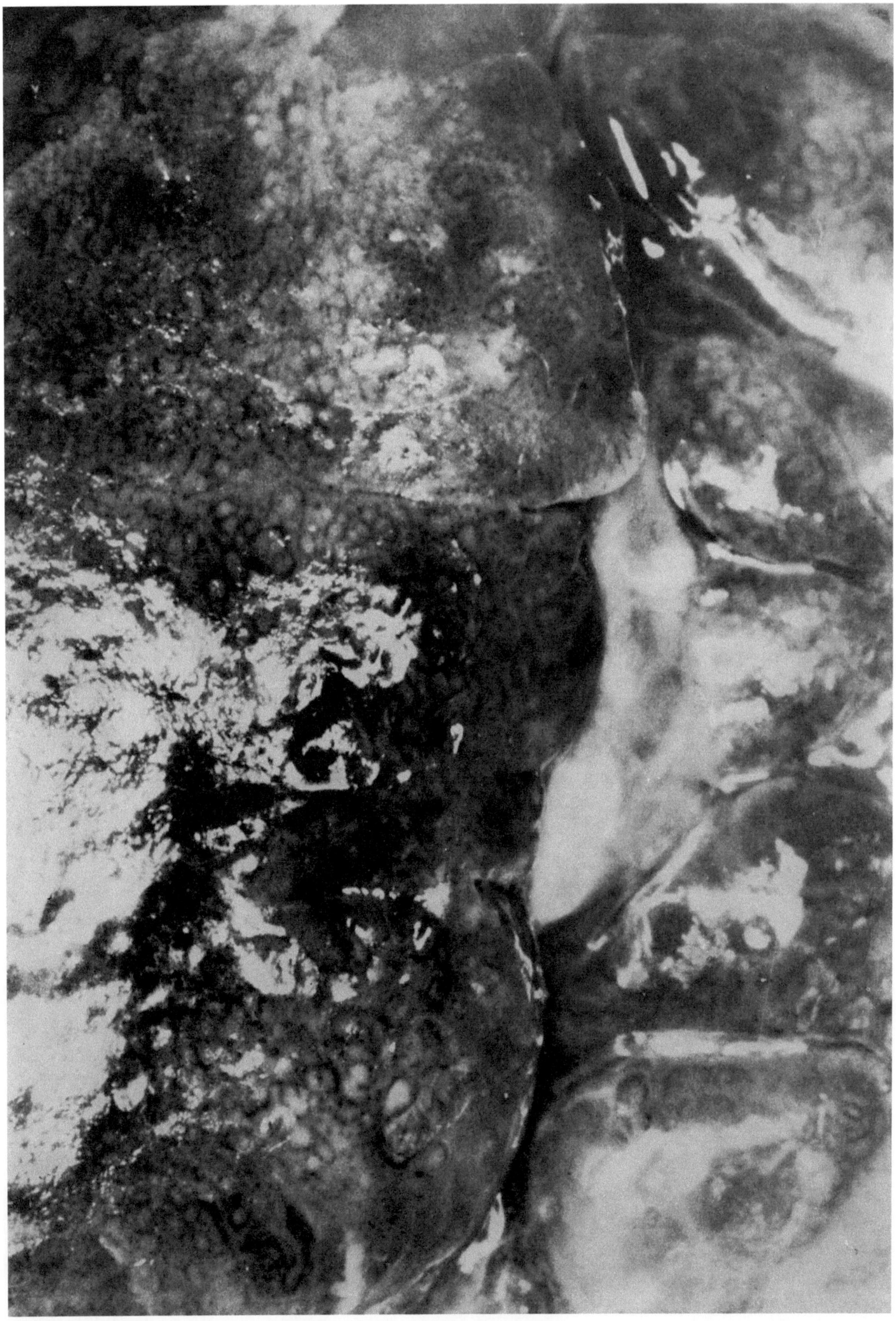

Plate 46 Mosaic

Scattered peaks of darker shade detectable from punctuated and partially keratinised field pattern with intercapillary spacings definitely enlarged and surface granular; moderate superficial keratinisation; colposcopic indication to presence of carcinoma in situ.

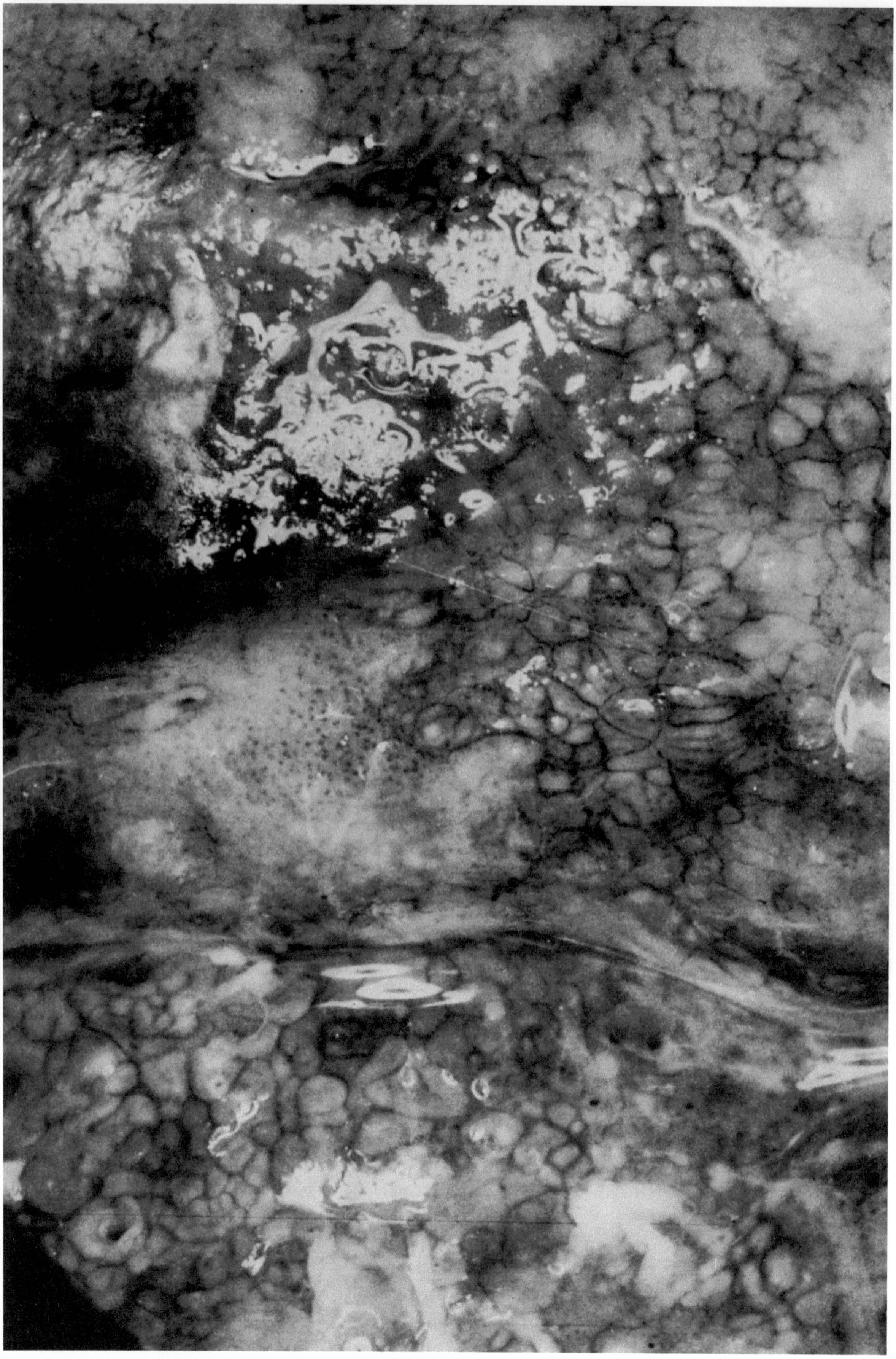

Plate 47 Mosaic, punctuation, keratosis, and invasive carcinoma

Bizarre keratinised field pattern with differences in level and increased trend to haemorrhage alternating with papillary floor regions; colposcopic representation of invasive carcinoma.

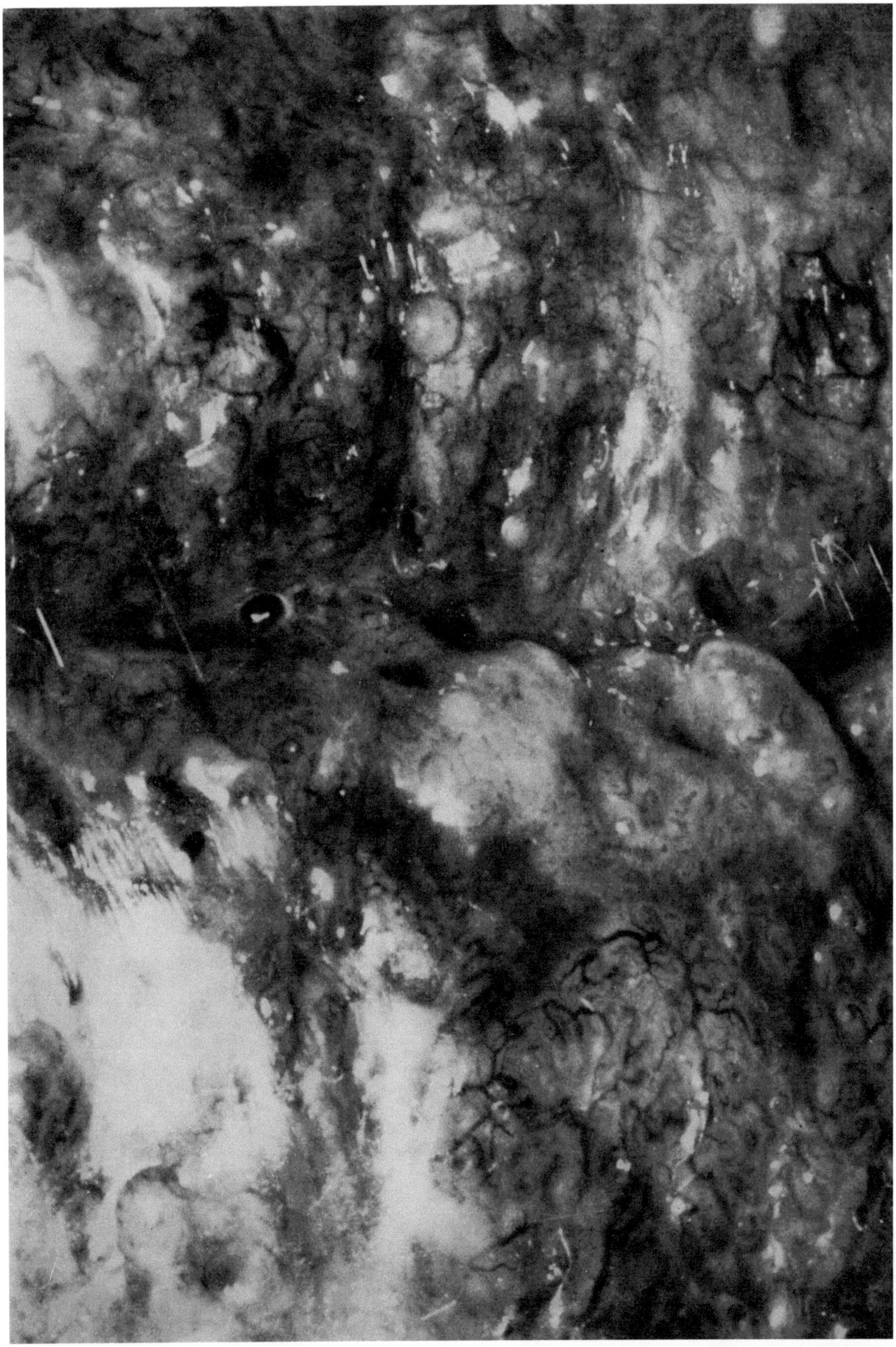

Plate 48 **Atypical vessels, invasive carcinoma**

Atypical carcinoma vessels with residues of network structure at anterior labium of os uteri; clearly washed-out carcinoma structures at posterior labium of os uteri.

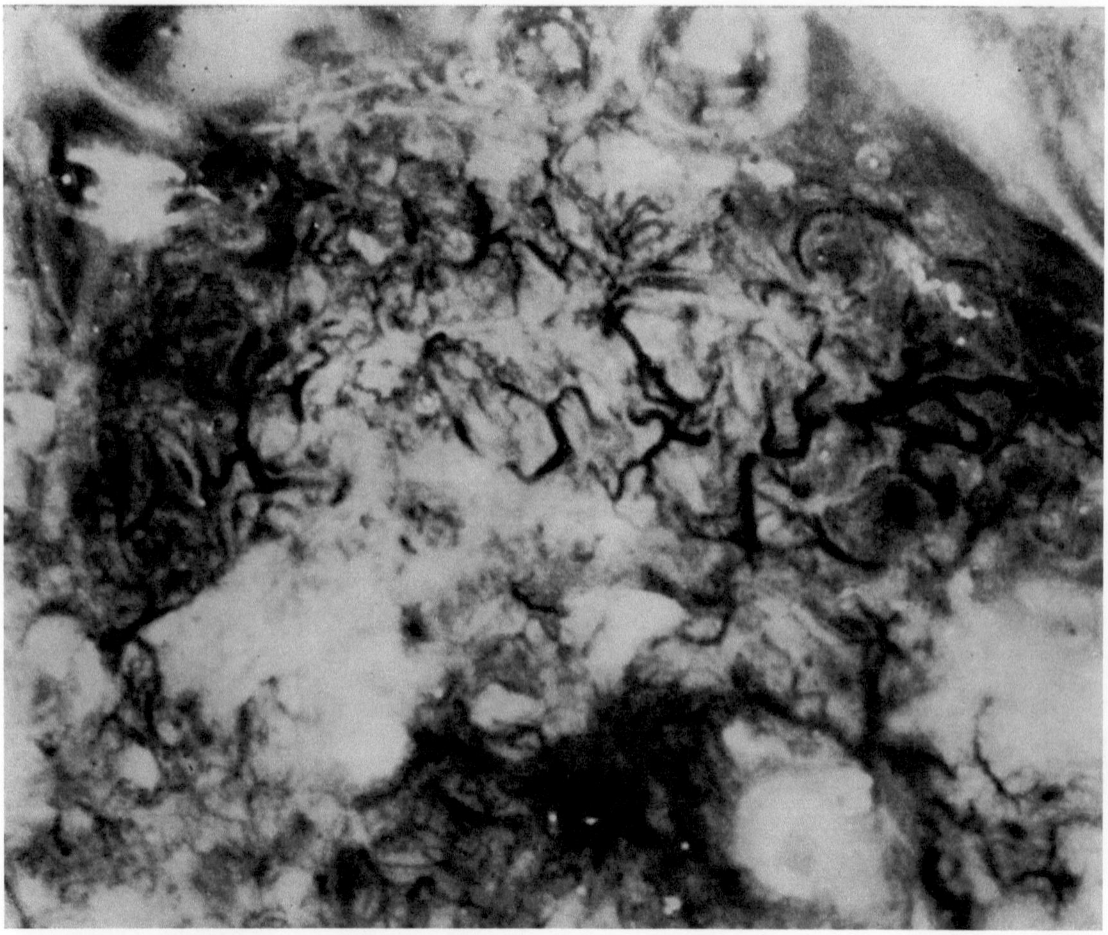

Plate 49 Atypical vessels, invasive carcinoma

Clearly atypical ramification vessels which, by all accounts and criteria, provide evidence to presence of invasive carcinoma (compare with normal ramification vessels of transformation zone).

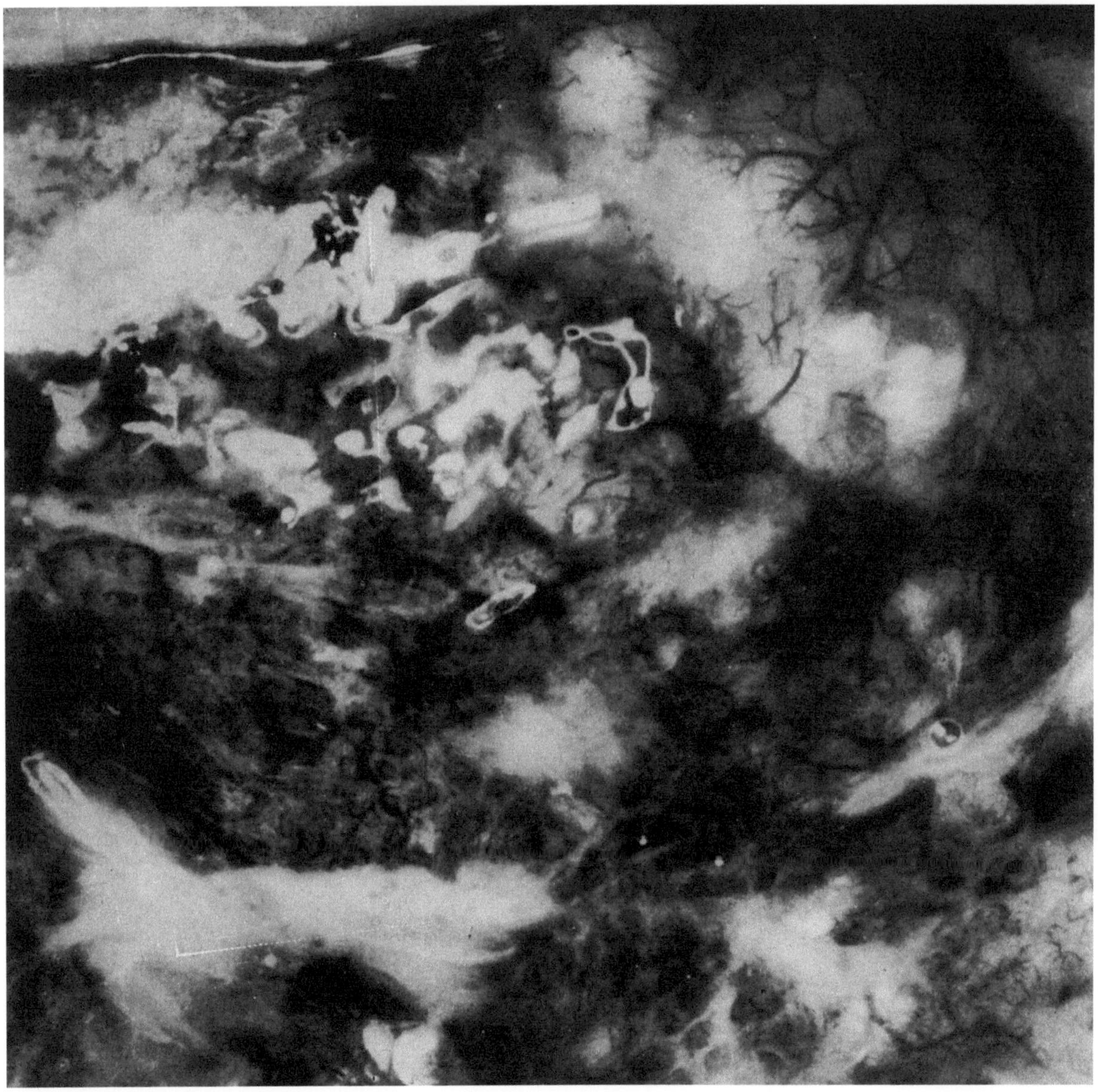

Plate 50 Mosaic, keratosis, atypical vessels

Washed-out appearance of carcinoma adjacent to relatively large negative field pattern area; ruptured bizarre carcinoma vessels and small regions of keratinisation in carcinoma centre; normal ramification vessels of closed transformation zone with epithelial atrophy depicted in right upper part of Plate.

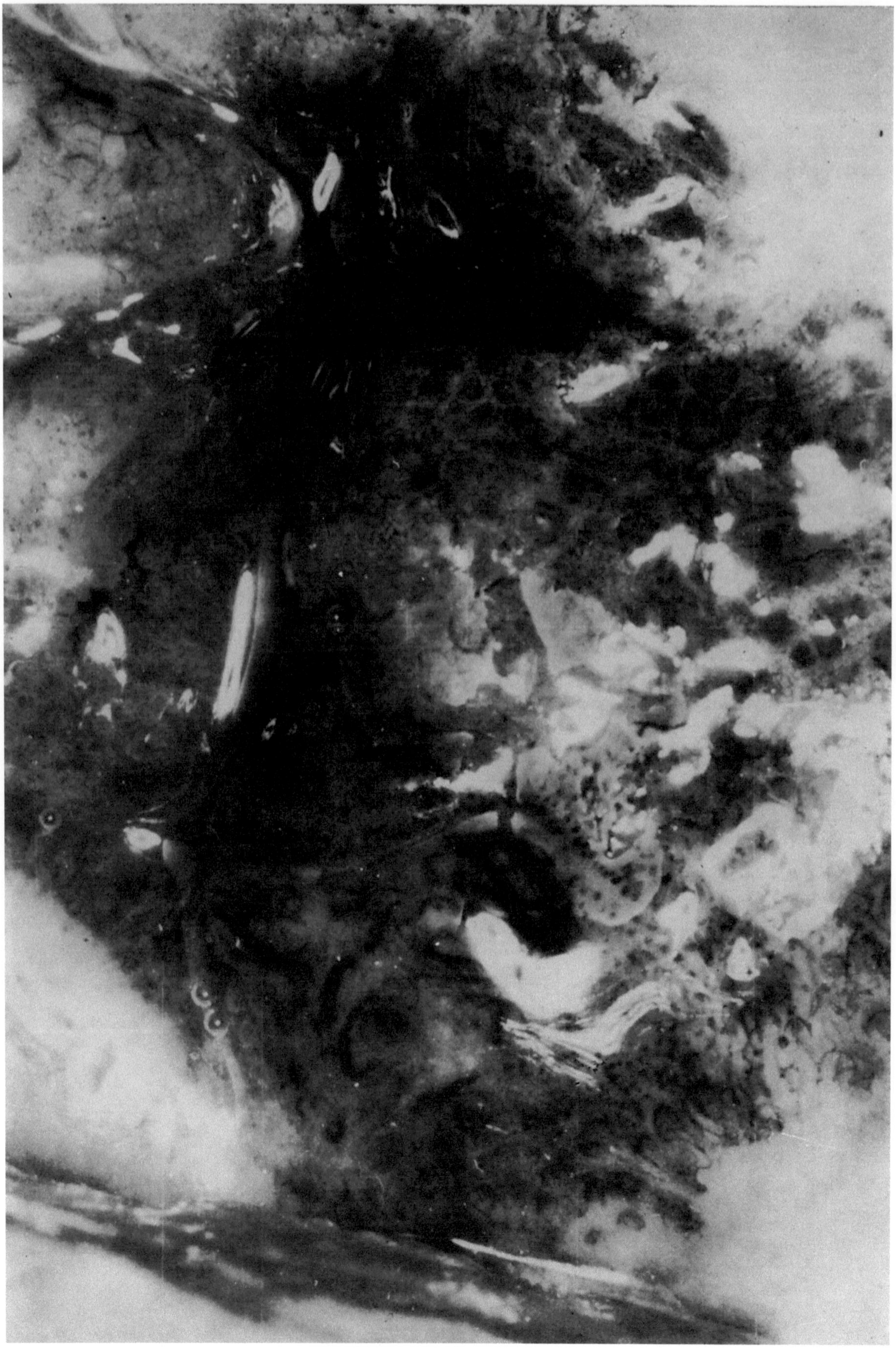

Plate 51 **Punctuation, mosaic, and carcinoma**

Negative field pattern areas in lower part of Plate and atypical hairpin capillaries in two upper thirds with continued stepwise degeneration and extending up to carcinoma.

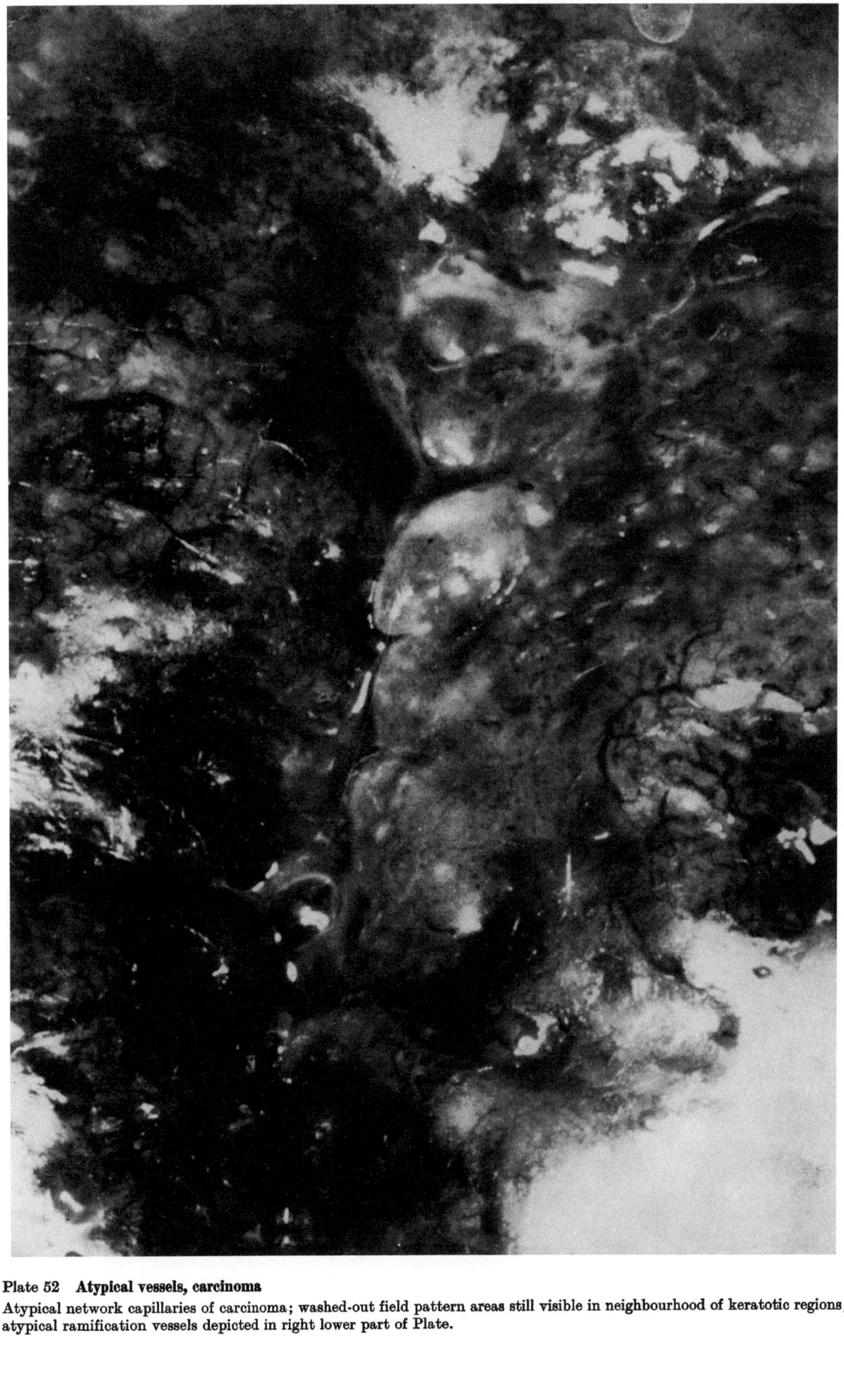

Plate 52 Atypical vessels, carcinoma

Atypical network capillaries of carcinoma; washed-out field pattern areas still visible in neighbourhood of keratotic regions; atypical ramification vessels depicted in right lower part of Plate.

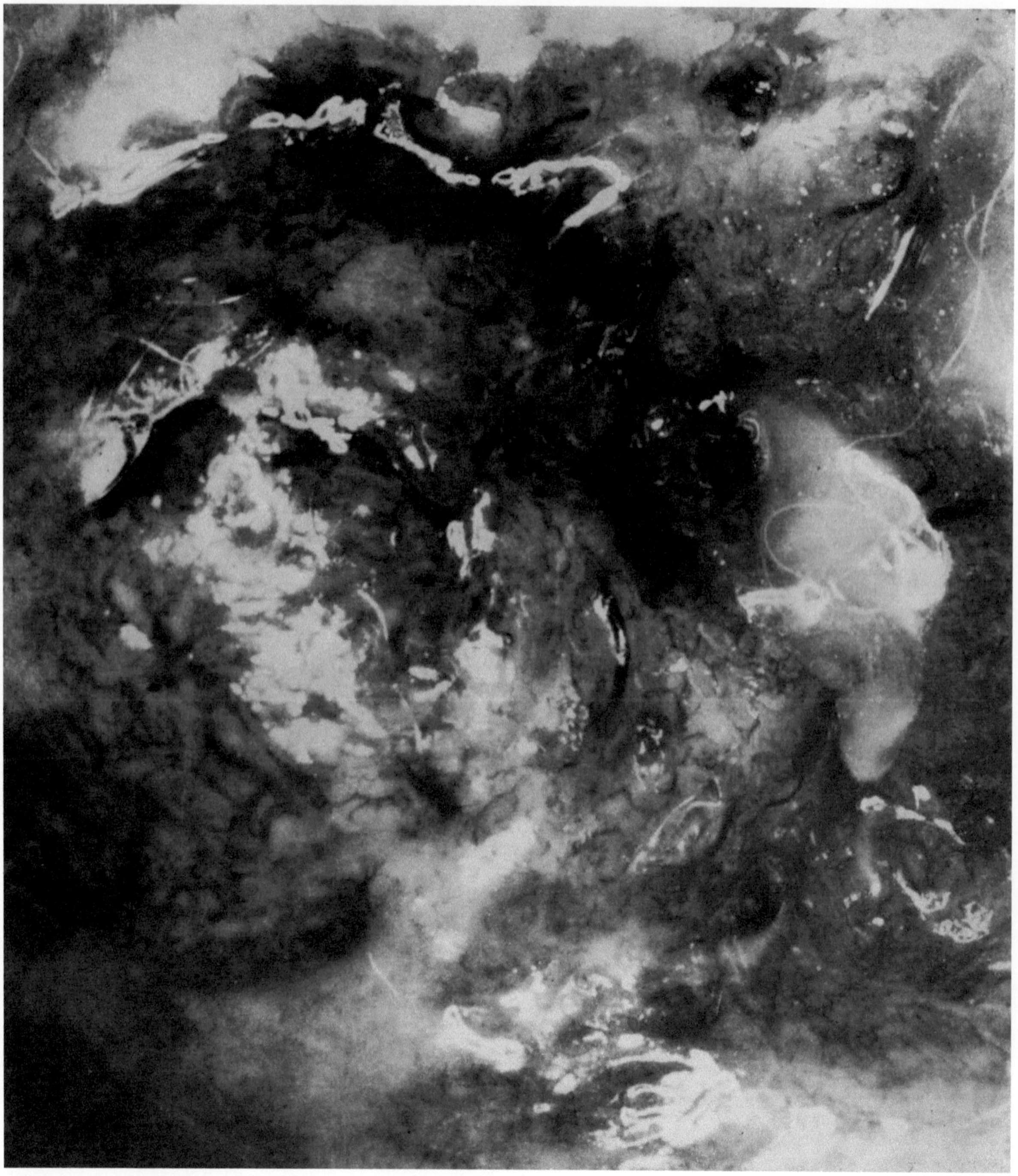

Plate 53 Atypical vessels
Atypical network vessels of exophytically growing invasive carcinoma.

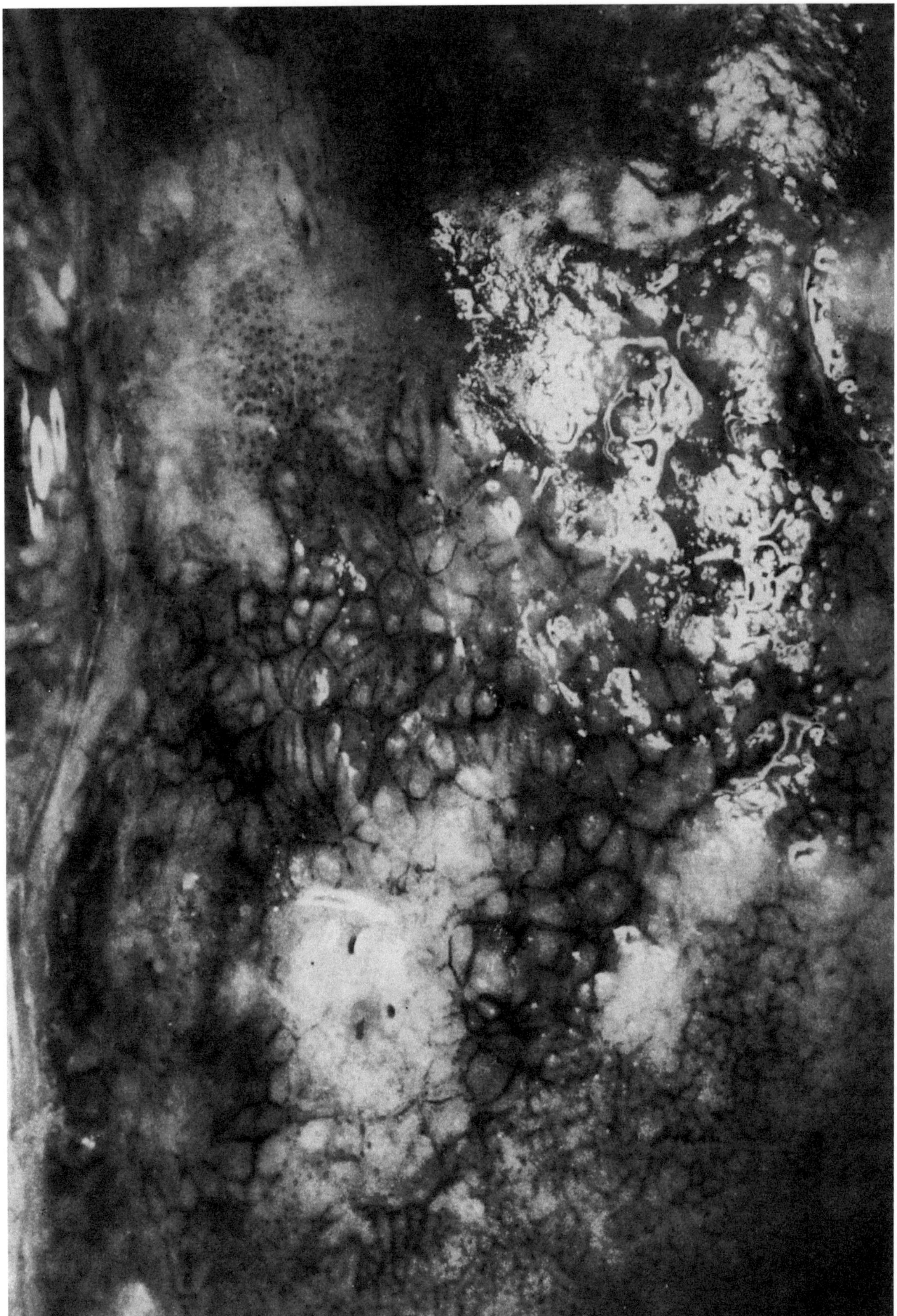

Plate 54 **Mosaic, punctuation, early invasive carcinoma**

Predominant appearance of atypical network vessels of simple field pattern, bizarre field pattern, and keratinised field pattern; atypical hairpin capillaries of papillary floor; no assessment possible of vascular structure on site of highest atypia in right upper part of Plate.

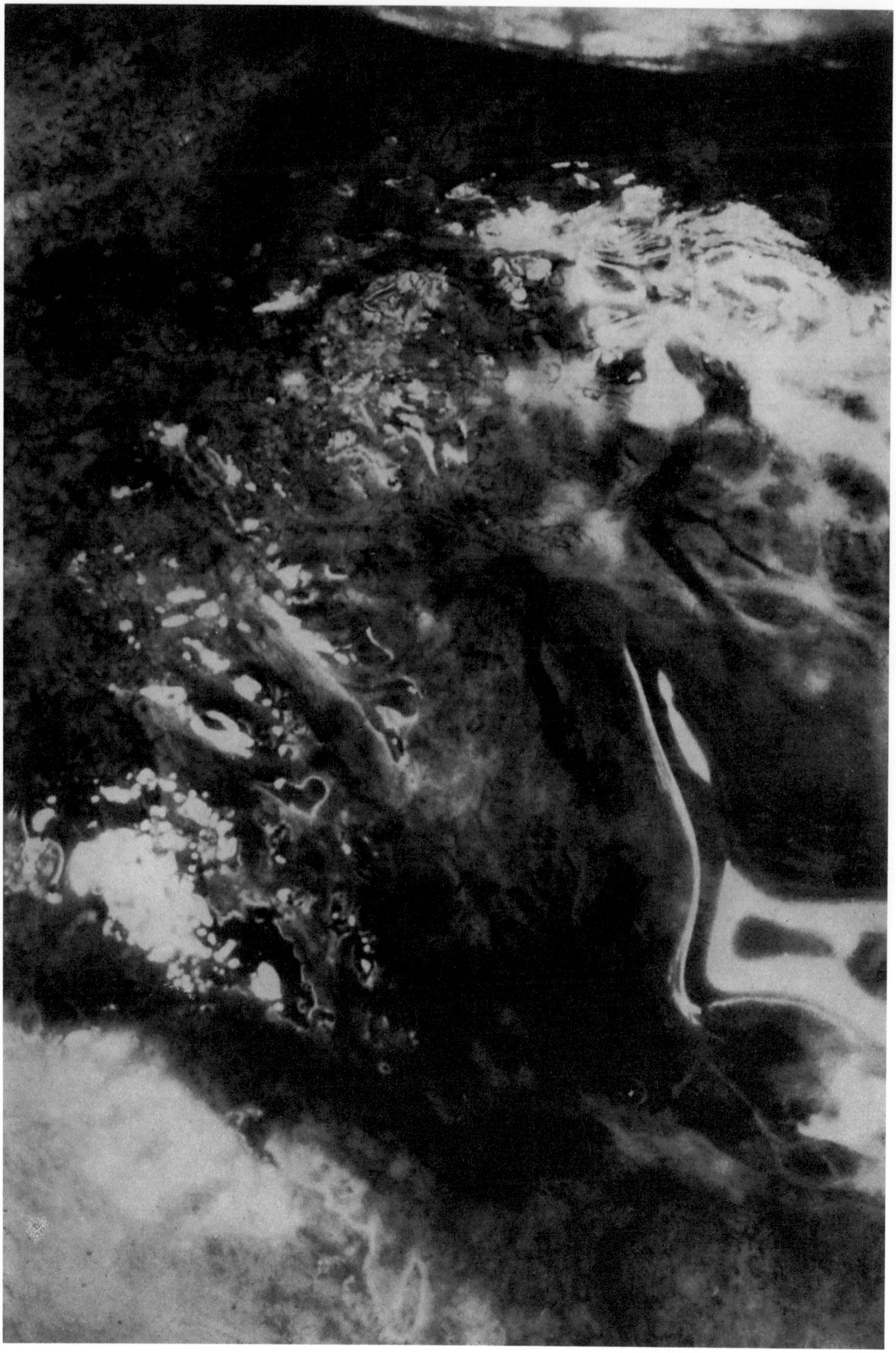

Plate 55 Atypical vessels, invasive carcinoma

Atypical carcinoma vessels, reminding of atypical network capillaries, together with epithelial defects and subepithelial bleeding of invasive carcinoma.

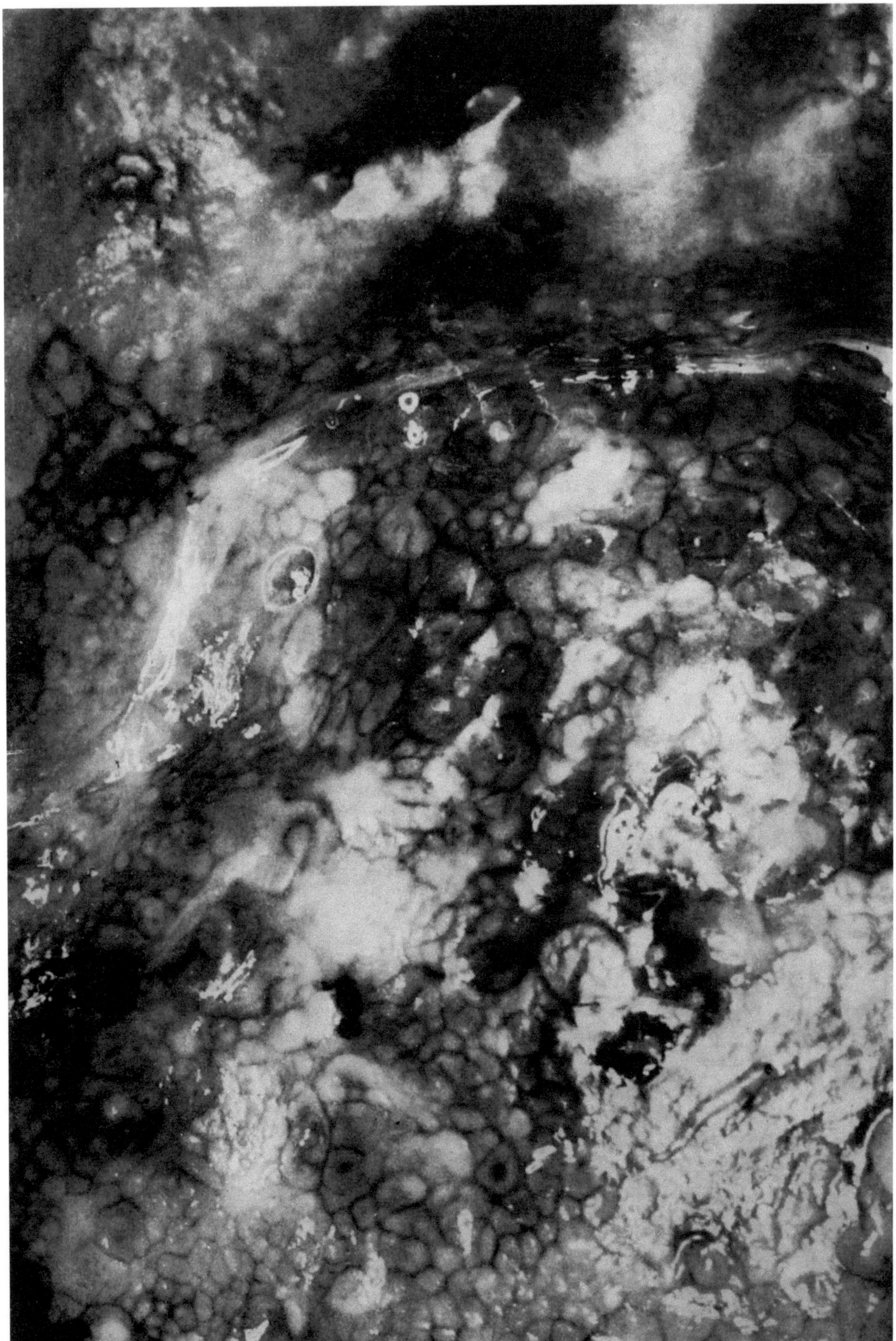

Plate 56 **Mosaic, keratosis, early invasive carcinoma**
Bizarre keratinised field pattern, strongly pronounced differences in level, and subepithelial haemorrhage; representation of early invasive carcinoma.

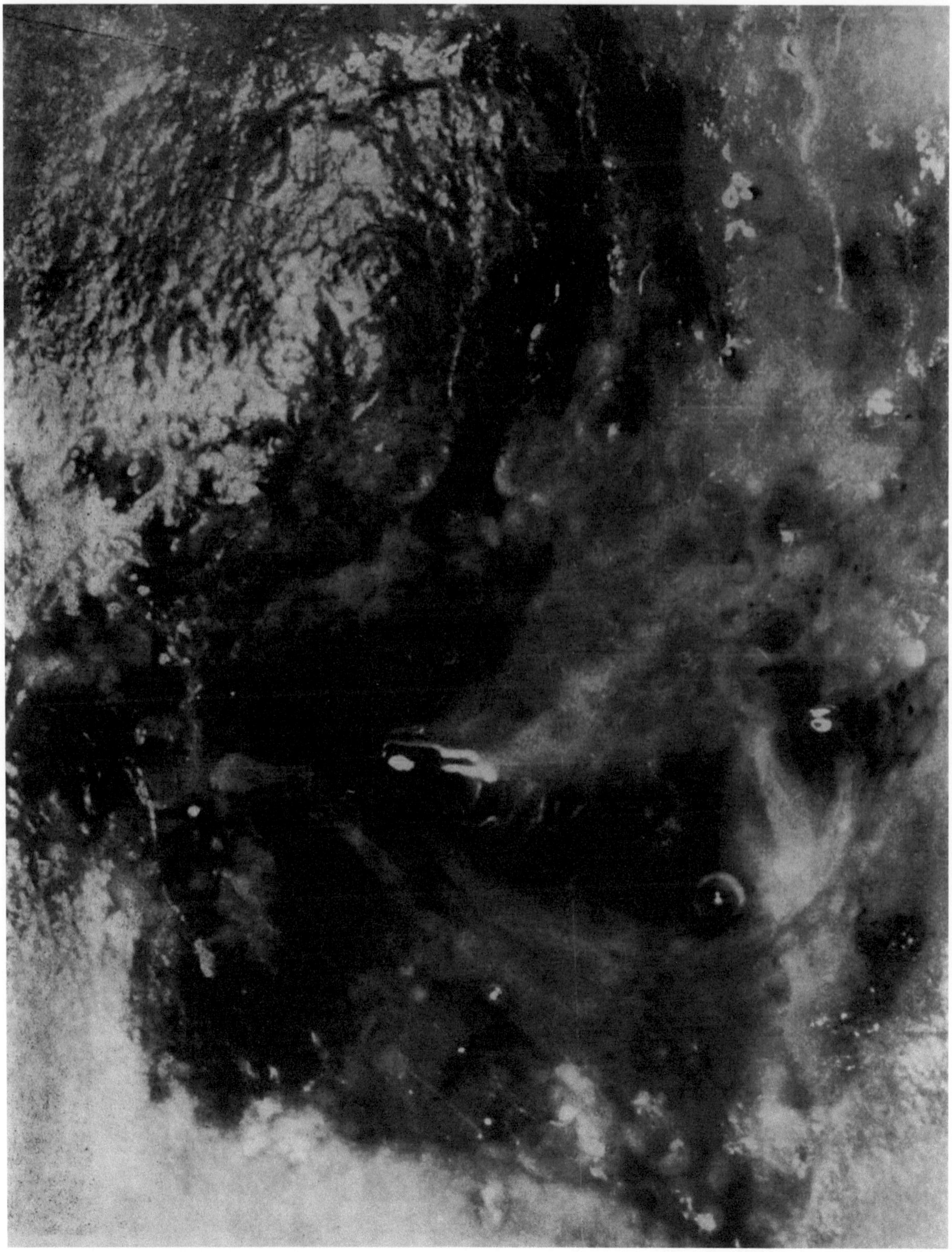

Plate 57 Mosaic, punctuation, and keratosis
The three most substantive manifestations of atypia of portio epithelium; trend to epithelial keratinisation may be accompanied by appearance of field pattern and floor with keratinisation or without; in extreme cases simple fields no longer identifiable as fields but resembling leucoplakia.

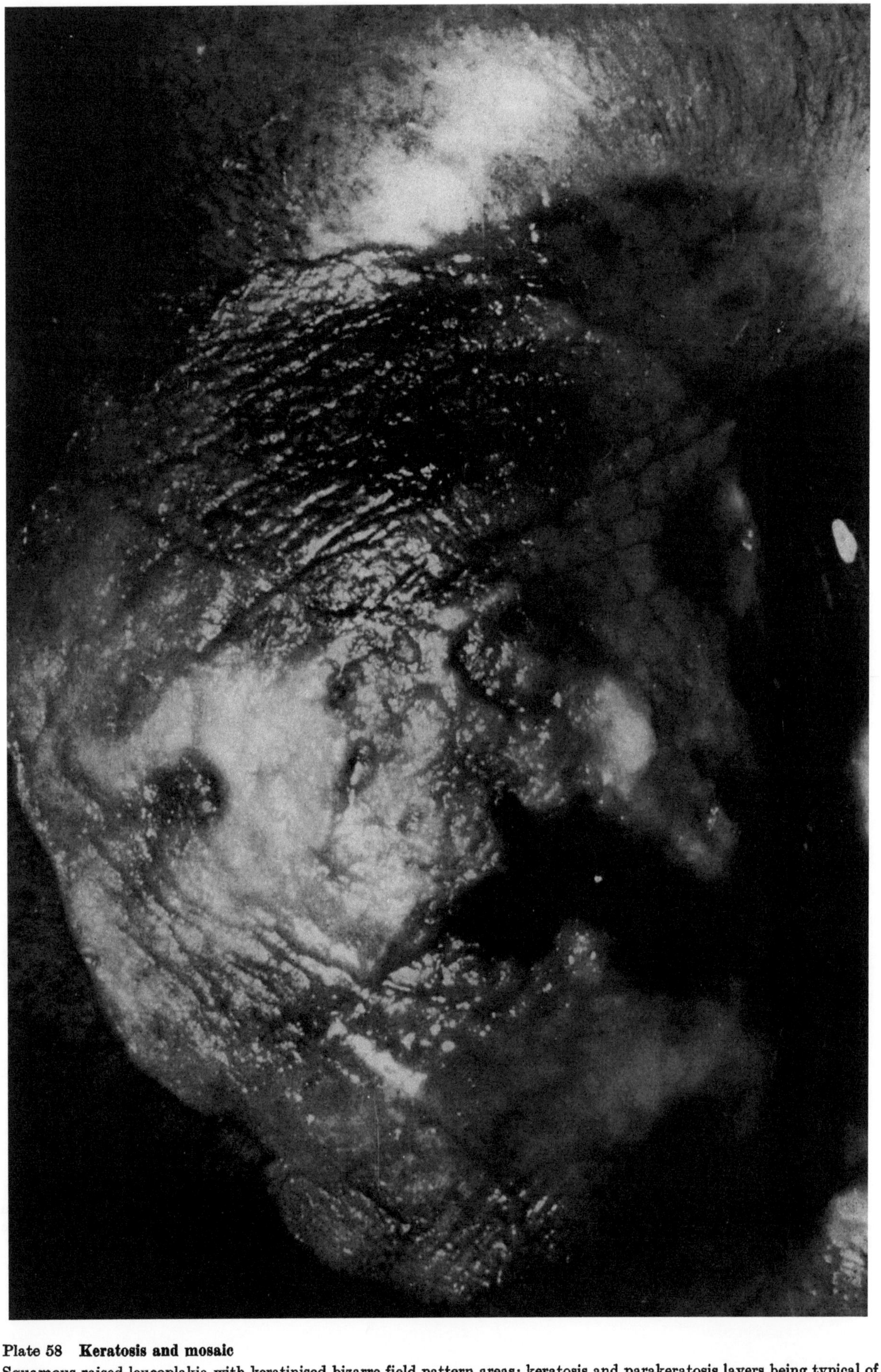

Plate 58 **Keratosis and mosaic**

Squamous raised leucoplakia with keratinised bizarre field pattern areas; keratosis and parakeratosis layers being typical of atypical epithelium under given conditions; thick, squamous, ruptured keratinised layers superimposed and suggesting occurrence of tough field pattern; atypical epithelium, colposcopically resembling floor or field pattern, recordable from underneath leucoplakia; leucoplakia often concealing presence of carcinoma, as in this case.

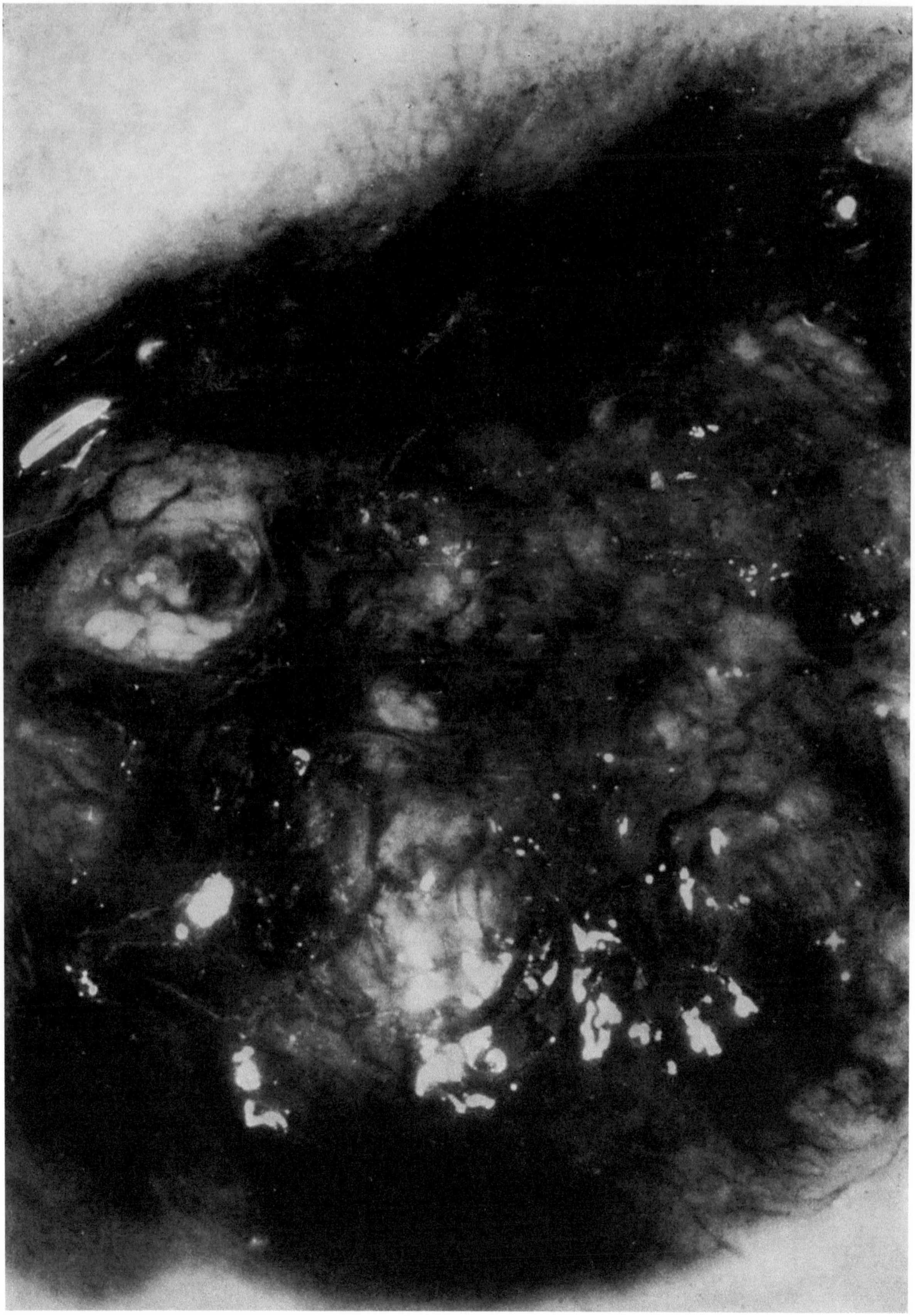

Plate 59 Macrocarcinoma

Tender field pattern structures still recognisable at anterior labium of os uteri, but exophytically growing tumour with car cinoma vessels of atypical network and ramification structures recordable from posterior labium of os uteri.

Vascular Patterns

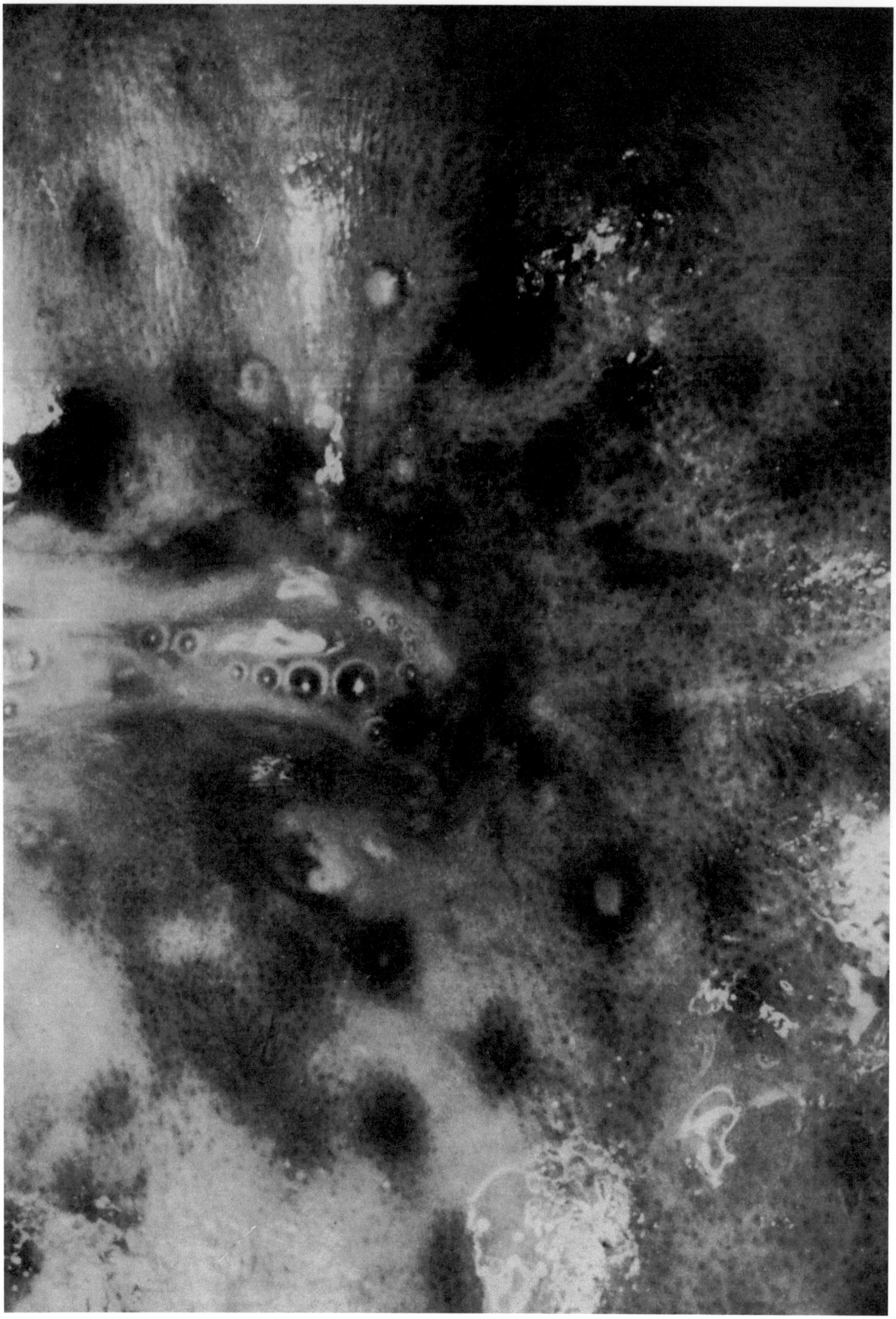

Plate 60 Inflammation

Normal hairpin capillaries of spotted and granular colpitis; conspicuous "double crests" of hairpin capillaries on the right side, as described primarily in context of trichomoniasis; distinctly restricted punctuation-floor areas must be delimited from such inflammatory processes by differential diagnosis; intercapillary spacings, according to *Koller* and *Kolstad*, reduced in benign inflammation, but enlarged in malignant transformation.

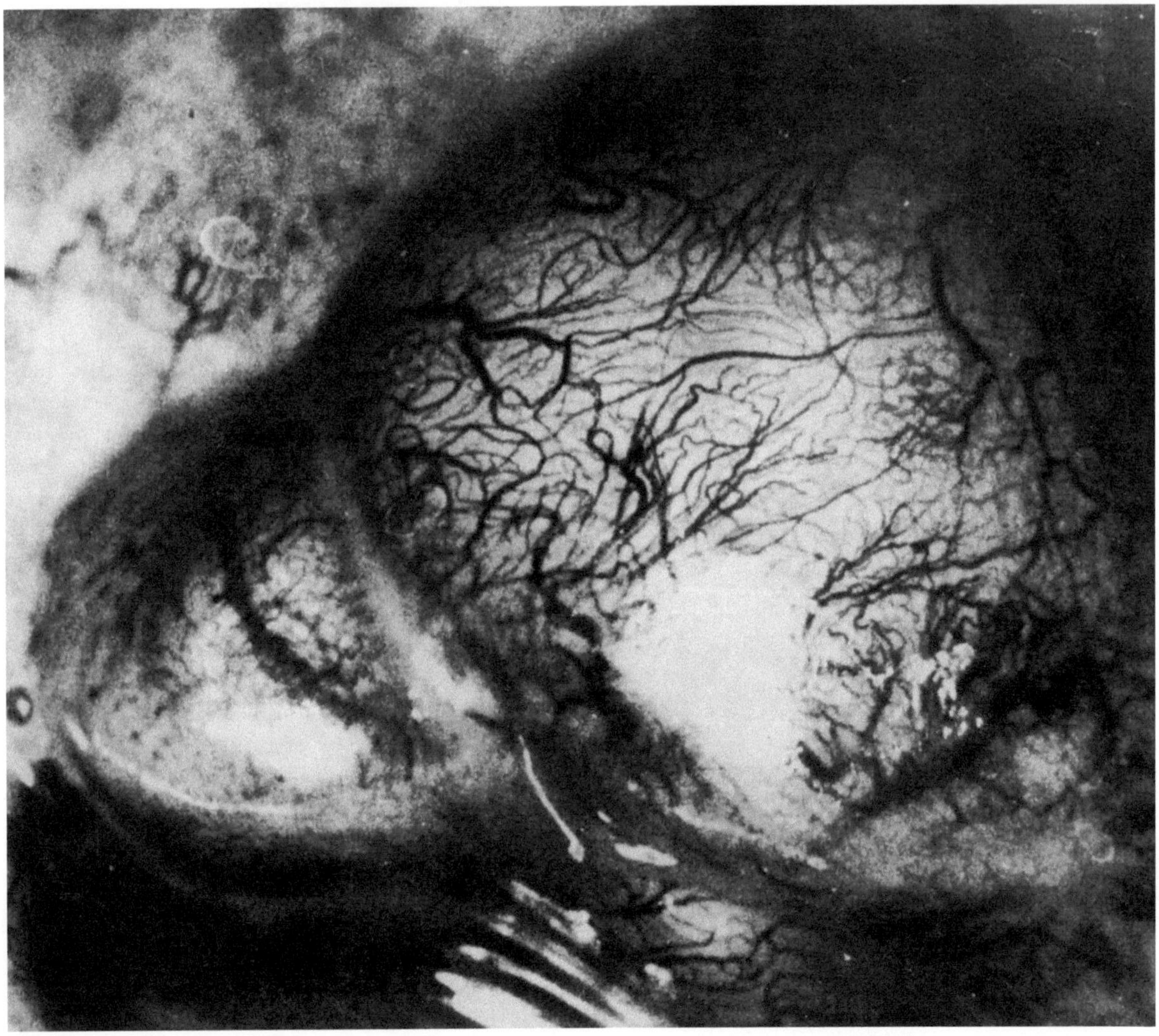

Plate 61 Transformation zone
Somewhat overlapping normal ramification vessels of closed transformation zone in region of Naboth's ovules.

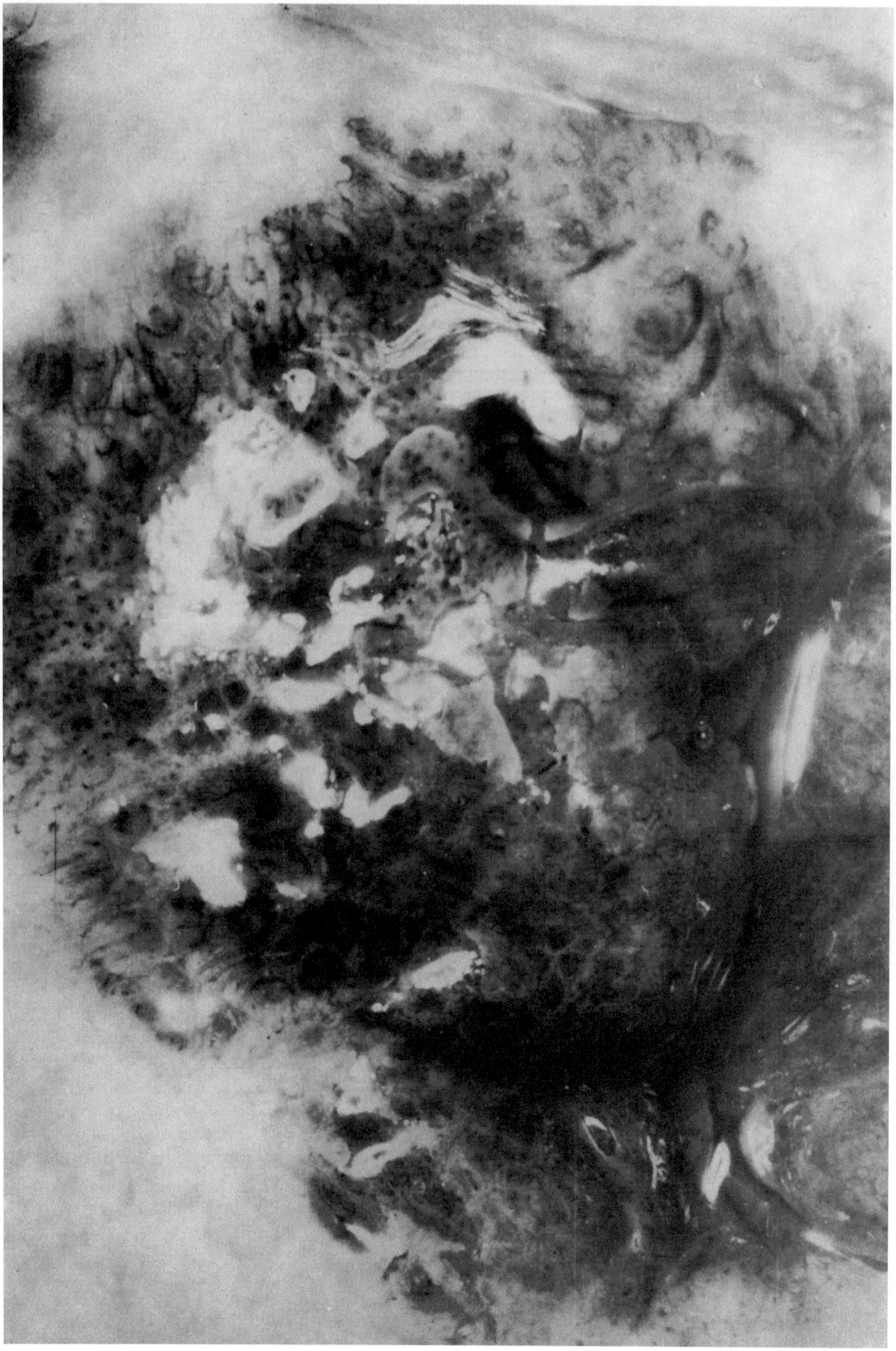

Plate 62 Mosaic, punctuation, atypical vessels

Irregular conglomeration of atypical hairpin vessels, scattered occurrence of long-drawn atypical vessels, comma-shaped vessels, and finest capillaries on top of negative field pattern, all being highly variegated and irregular, typical of early invasive carcinoma.

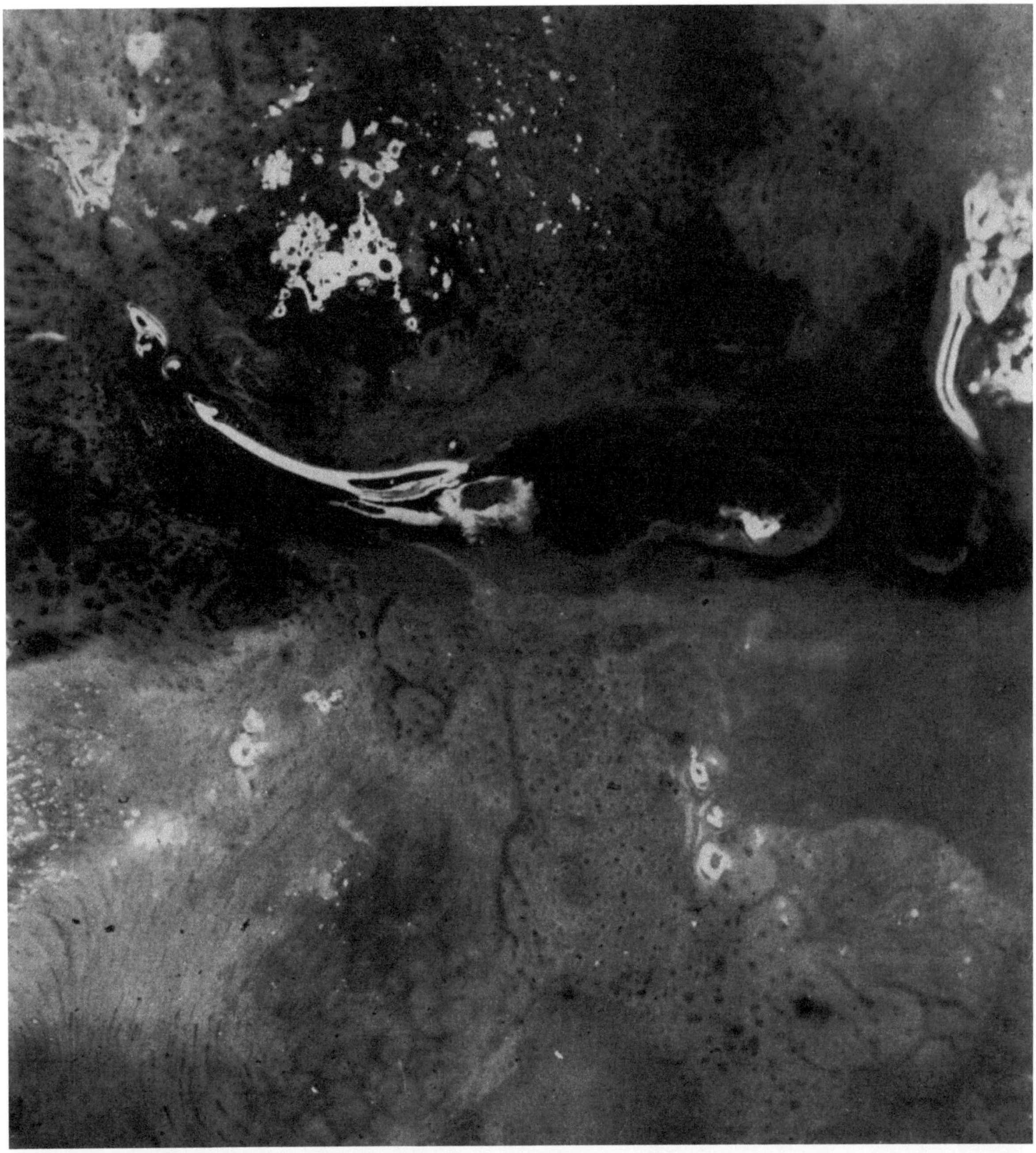

Plate 63 **Mosaic, punctuation, and atypical vessels**

Atypical hairpin capillaries of early invasive carcinoma accompanied by tender field pattern structures; areas of vessels comparable to those depicted in Plate 62 on anterior labium of os uteri; also visible are numerous spotted points of haemorrhage caused by fragility of vessels.

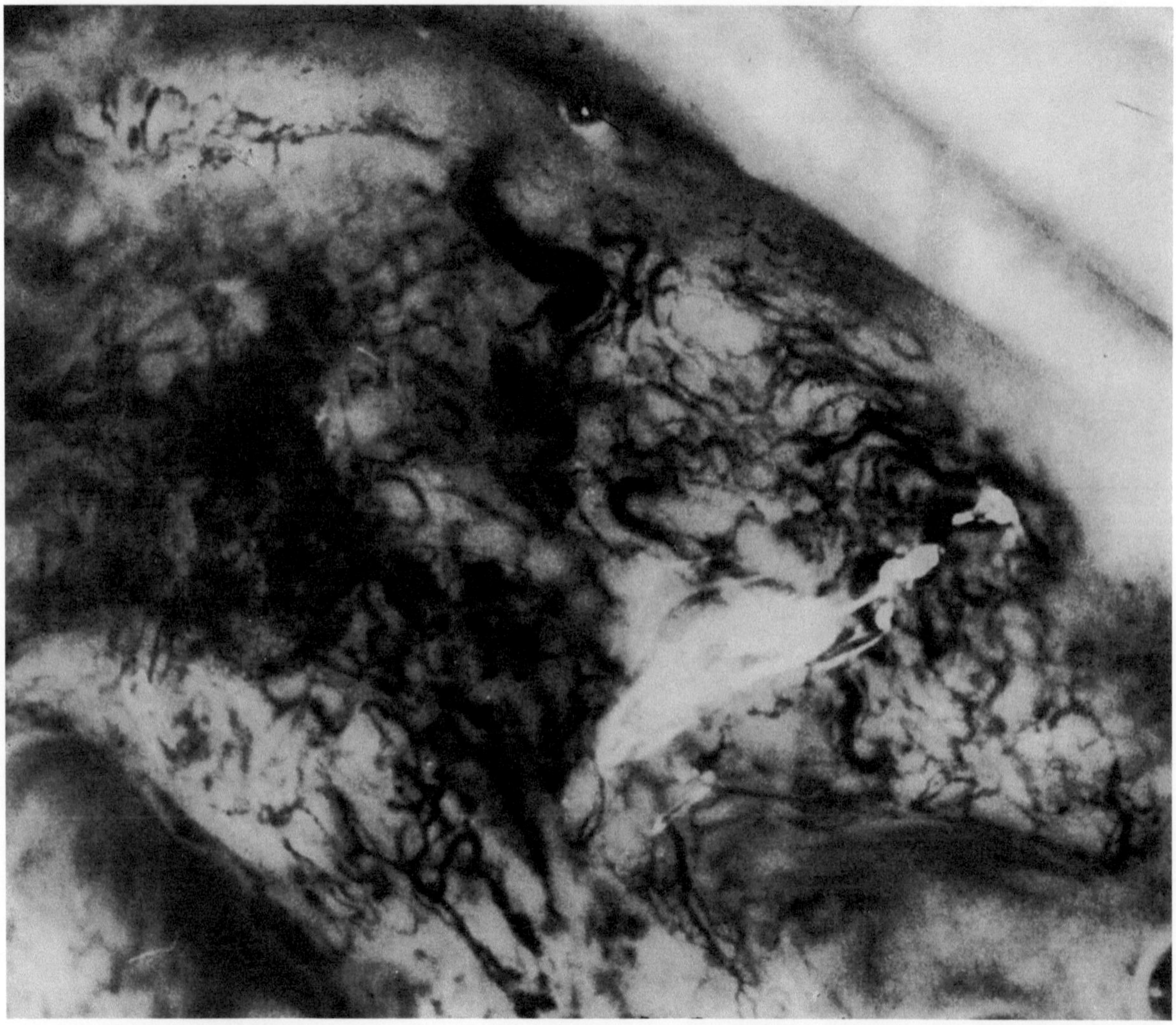

Plate 64 Atypical vessels and carcinoma

Atypical carcinoma vessels of network type: variation in size, shape, alignment, calibre, ruptures, and intercapillary spacings; confusion and irregularity of entire, vascular pattern.

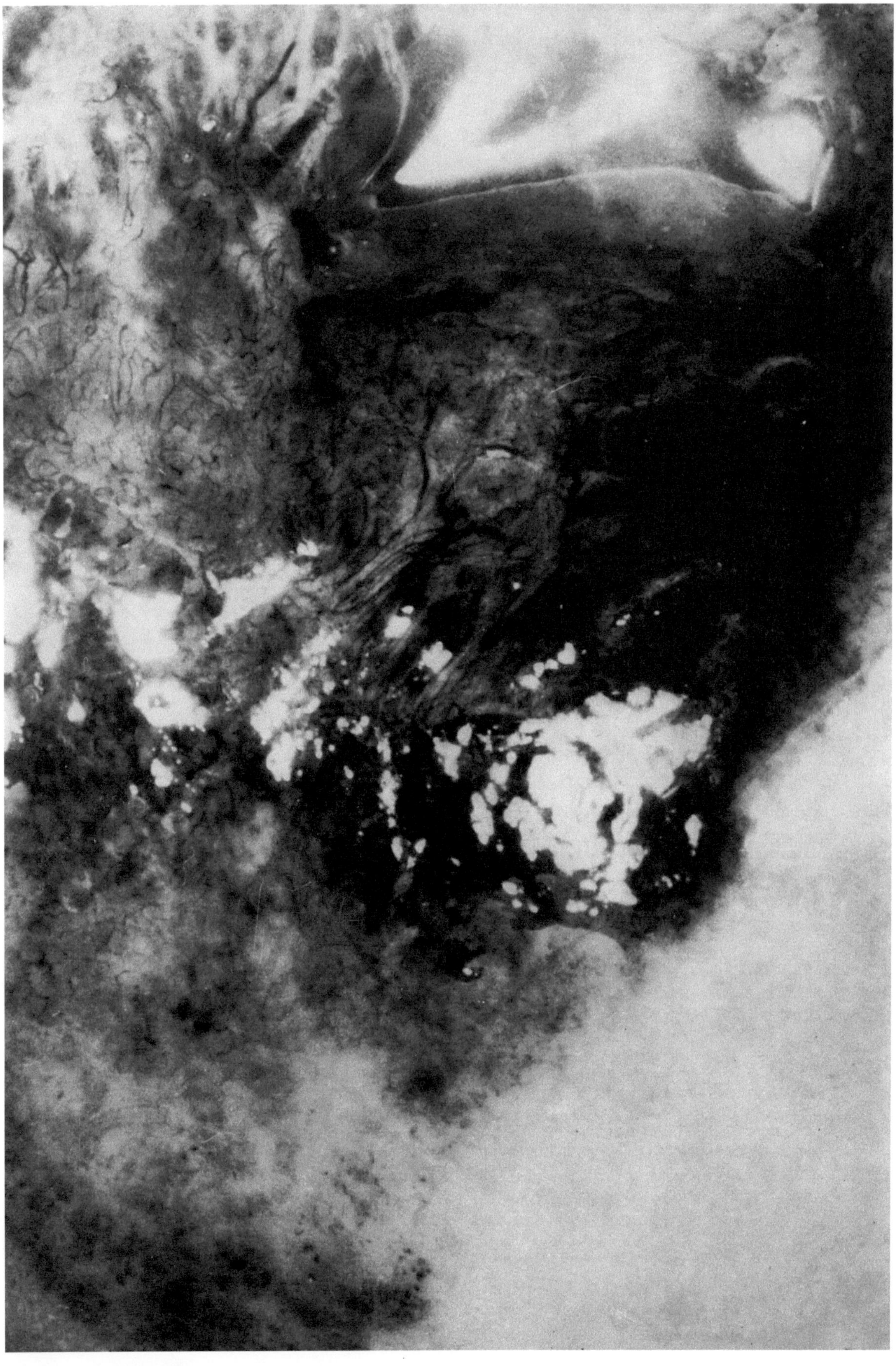

Plate 65 **Atypical vessels**
Finely shaped, sometimes parallel vessels together with comma-shaped vessels and atypical hairpin vessels being typical of early invasive carcinoma

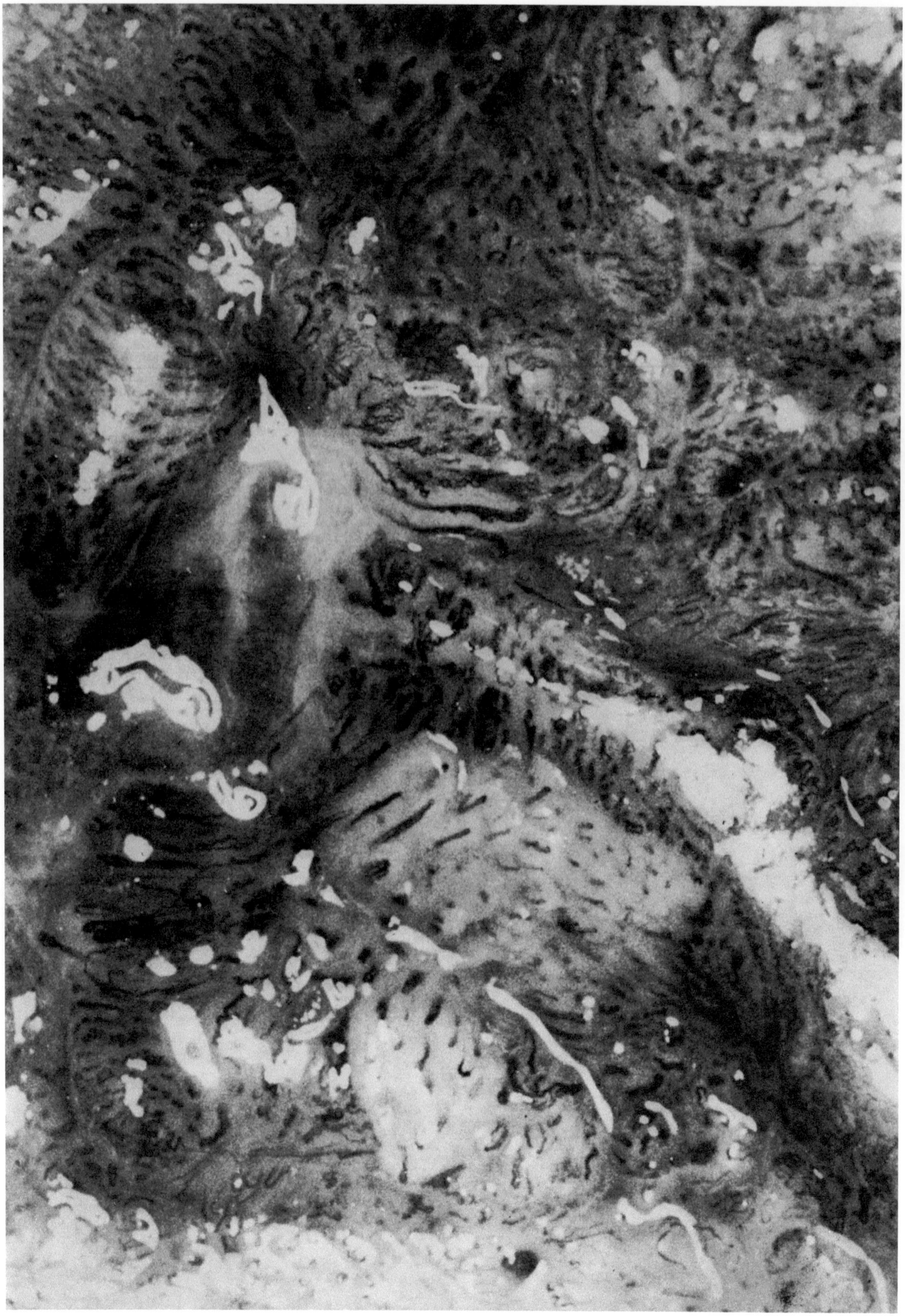

Plate 66 **Atypical vessels, carcinoma**

These atypical carcinoma vessels have originated from atypical hairpin capillaries; glomerulation, twisting, and calibre variation clearly visible by lateral view; conspicuous alternation of areas of high vascular density with areas of relative avascularity.

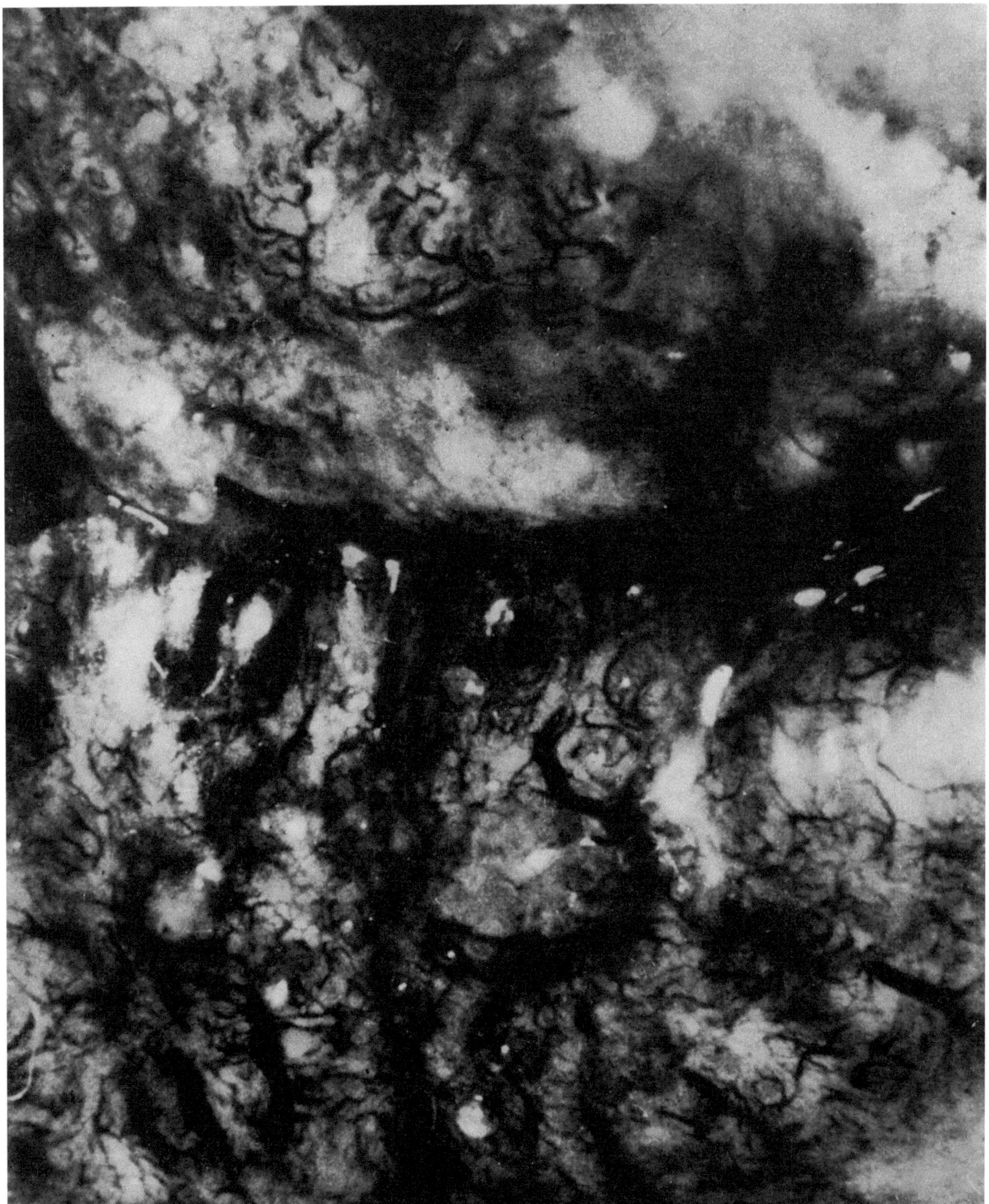

Plate 67 **Atypical vessels, carcinoma**

Atypical ramification vessels of invasive carcinoma on surface with exophytic nodular alteration; relatively easy to make straightforward diagnosis of ordinary carcinoma.

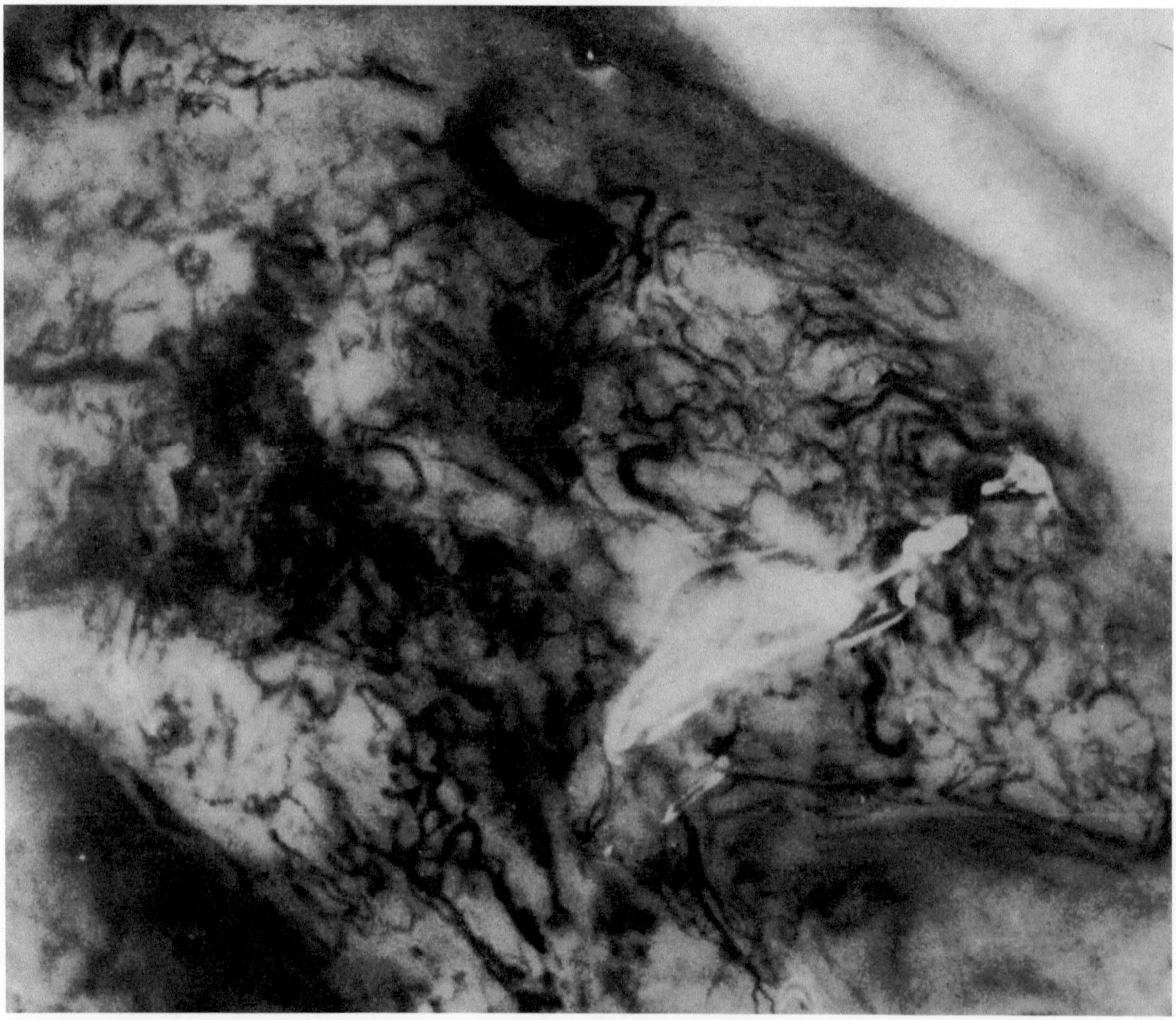

Plate 68 Atypical vessels, carcinoma
Atypical vascular pattern, originated from network type, in a case of ordinary carcinoma.

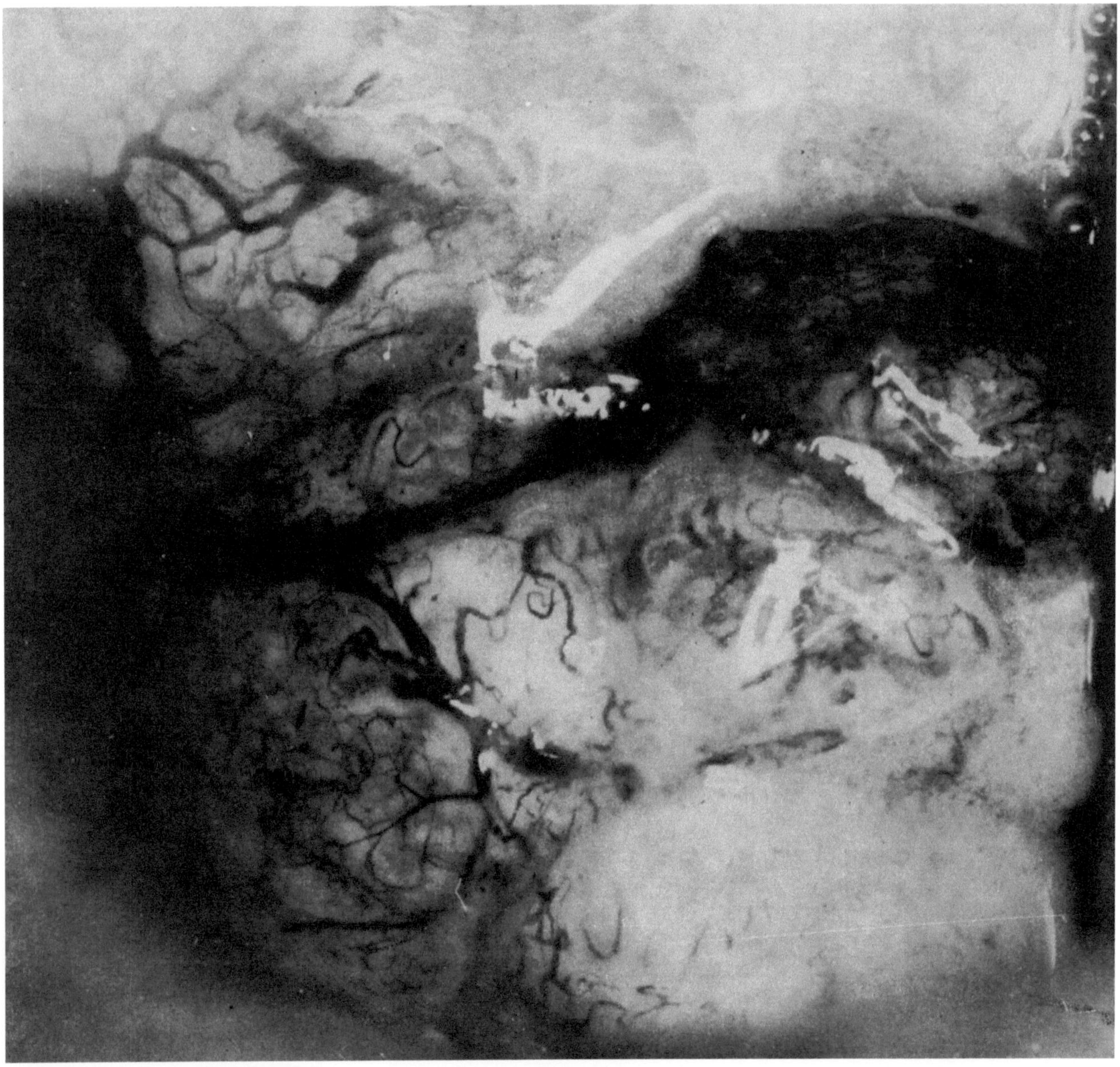

Plate 69 Atypical vessels, carcinoma
Atypical ramification vessels of macrocarcinoma of clearly bizarre angio-architecture of insufficient vascular system.

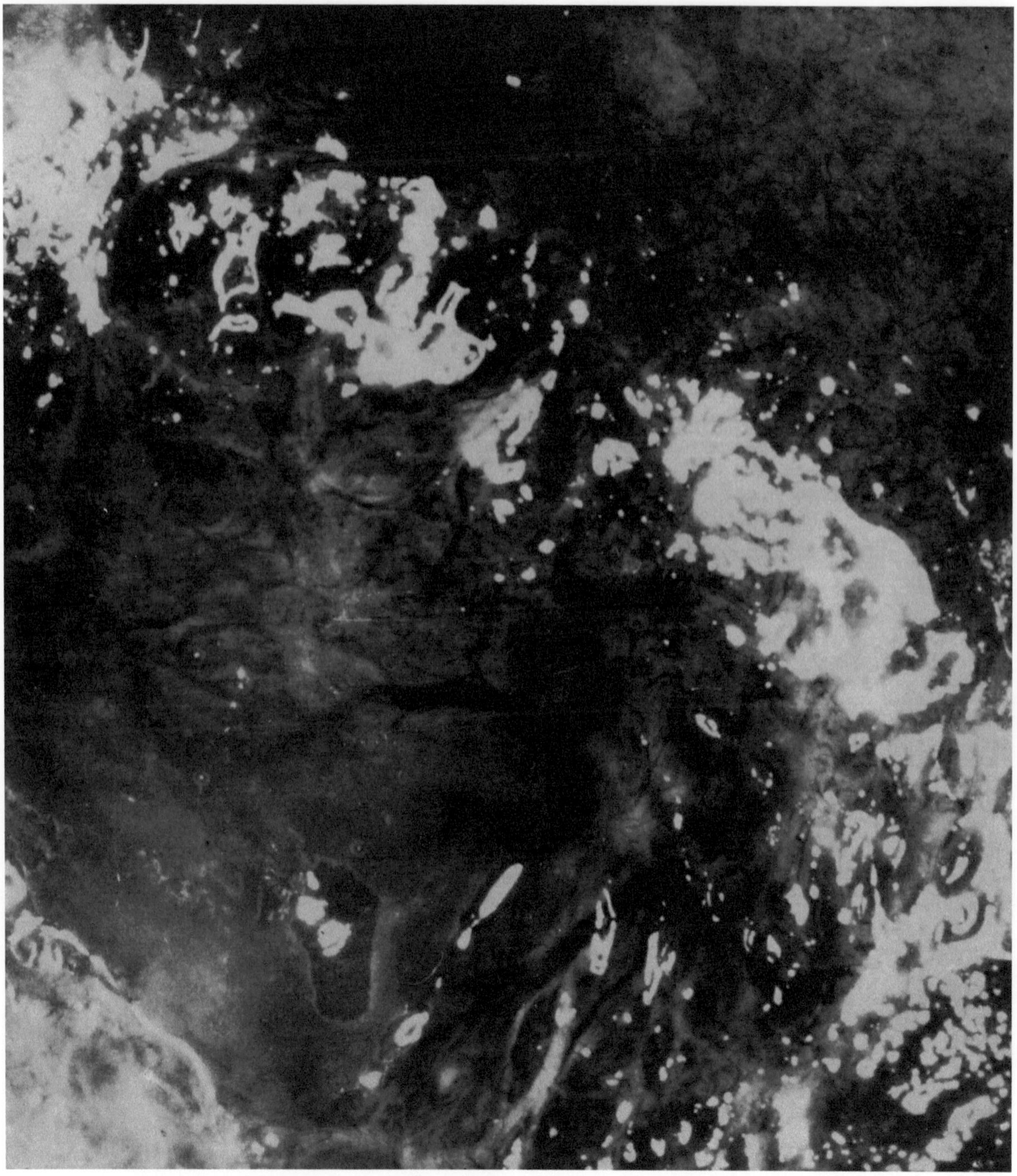

Plate 70 Atypical vessels, carcinoma
Predominance in this carcinoma of relatively densely arranged atypical network vessels, petechia, and difference in level of washed-out tissue.

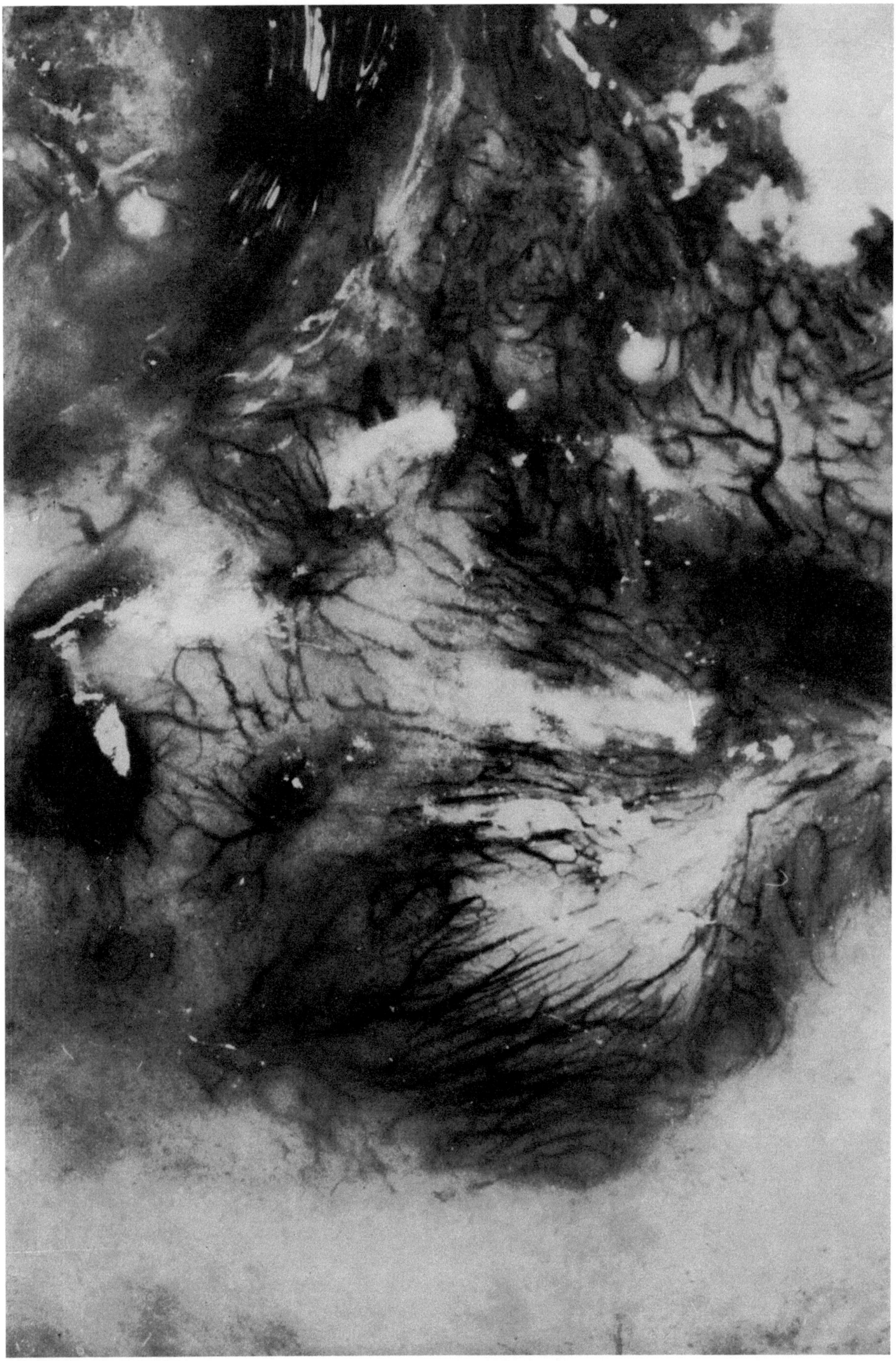

Plate 71 Atypical vessels
Elongated ramification vessels in rigid vascular structure; condition after irradiation of ordinary cervical carcinoma.

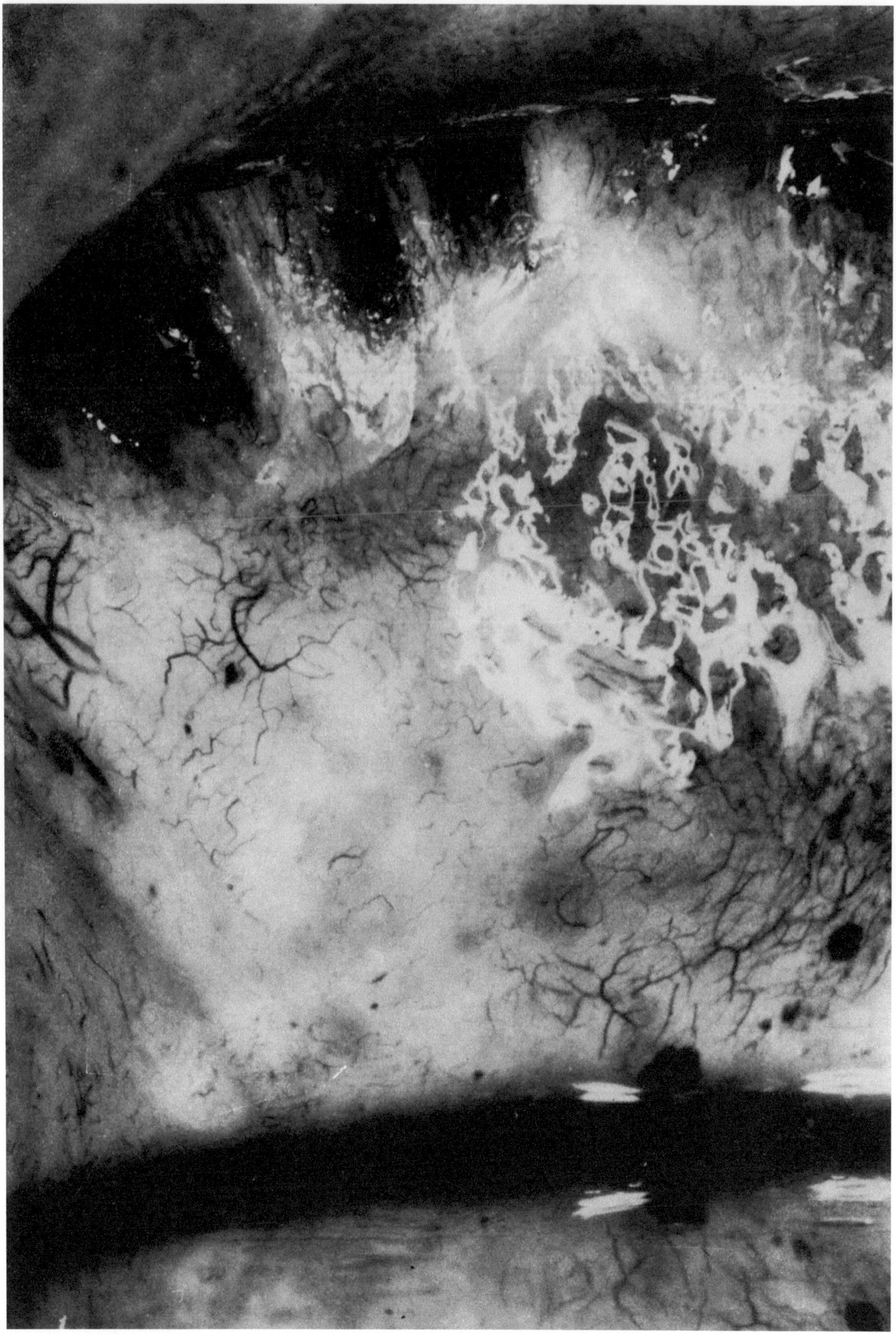

Platte 72 **Vascular pattern**

Widely normalised vascular pattern of carvical carcinoma, following successful radiotherapy; classical carcinoma vessels tend to undergo normalisation, within weeks and months, in response to radiotherapy; carcinomas not controllable by radiotherapy will not change their own carcinomatous vascular typicality (***Rieck***), whereas normalisation of vascular alignment may be interpreted as a sign of favourable prognosis.

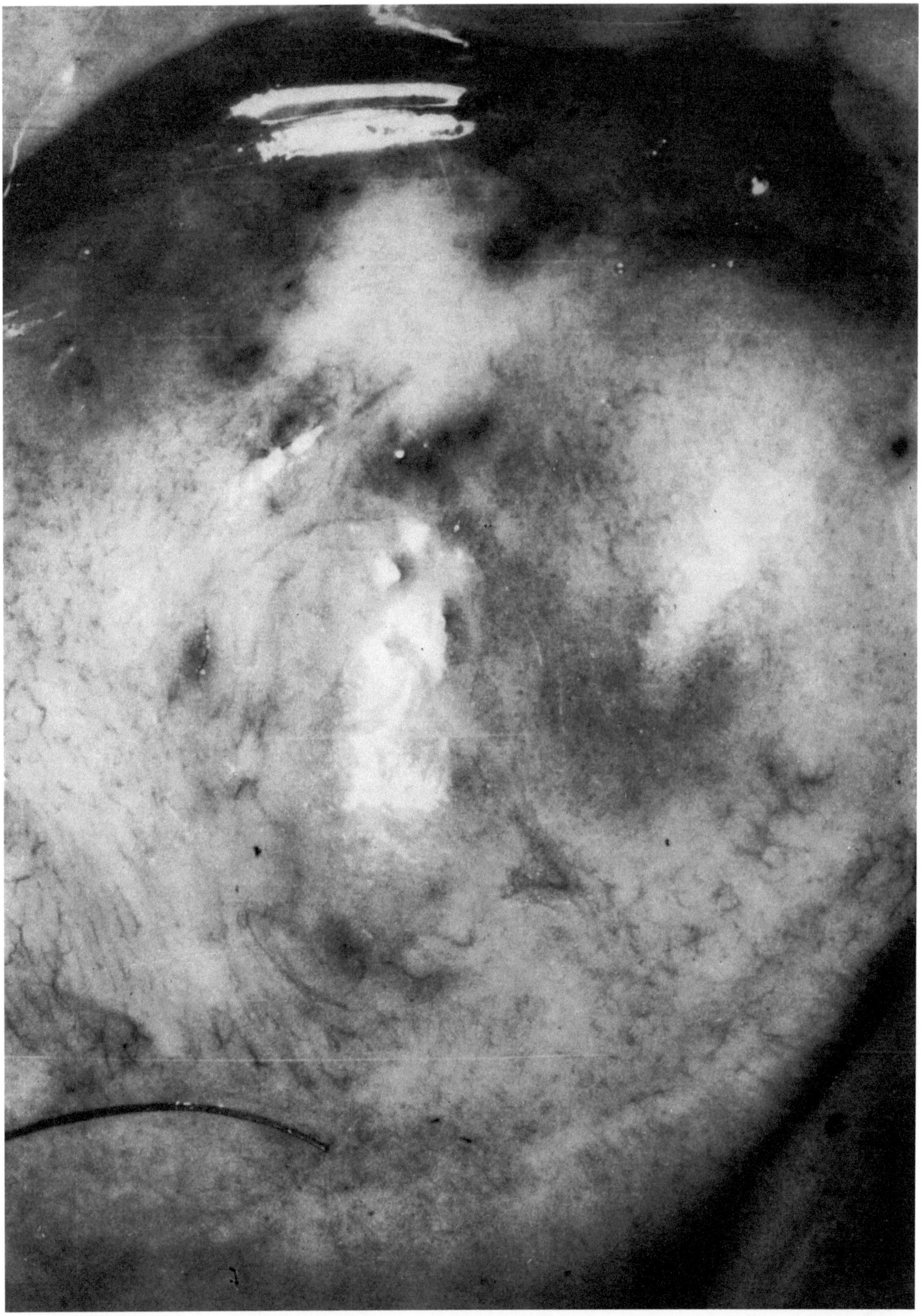

Plate 73 Vascular pattern
Widely normalised vascular pattern of early invasive cervical carcinoma, following successful specific chemotherapy (Rifampicin-*Eschbach*).